GOOD
FOOD
FOR
LIFE

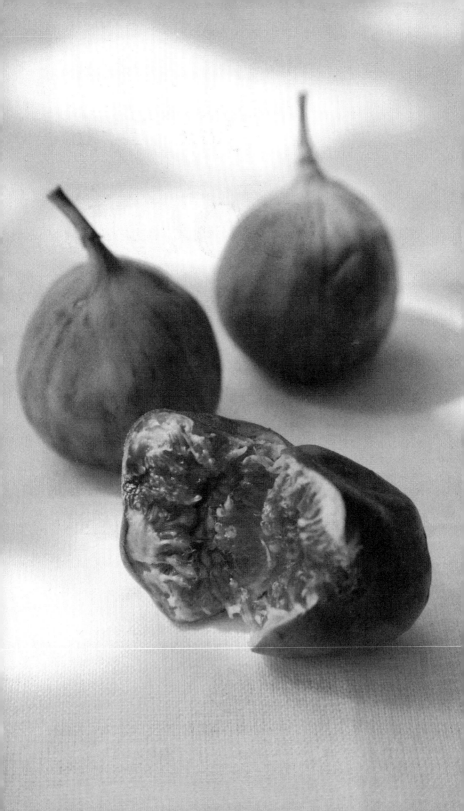

Jane Clarke

GOOD FOOD FOR LIFE

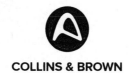

COLLINS & BROWN

To Maya

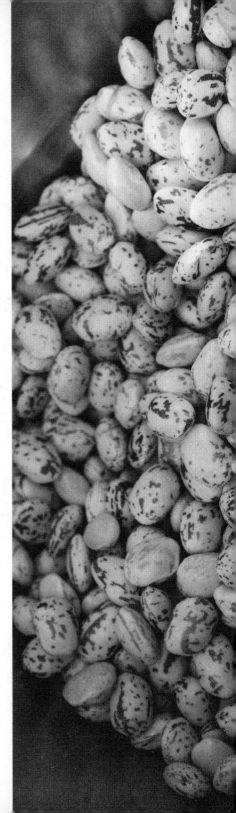

First published in the United Kingdom by
Collins & Brown
10 Southcombe Street
London W14 0RA

An imprint of Anova Books Company Ltd

ISBN 978-1-90939-776-7

A CIP catalogue for this book is available from the
British Library.

10 9 8 7 6 5 4 3 2 1

Printed and bound by Bookwell, Finland

This book can be ordered direct from the publisher
at www.anovabooks.com

Contents

Introduction

For me one of the driving forces (if not the major one) in setting up my practice over 15 years ago – where today I treat people ranging from young to old, through every stage of their lives – was realising that if we are to be able to nourish our bodies throughout our lifetime, the food has to be delicious. While one can stomach the odd mouthful of healthy gruel, or indeed get a bizarre buzz out of sticking to an abstemious, punishingly boring diet for a week or two, when it comes down to enjoying life, we need to find foods that are easy, inspiring and scrumptious.

This is the job I love: turning life around for people who have lost their way with eating or who have found themselves in a situation where their body is struggling. It's not about being a holier-than-thou puritan food faddist who is everyone's worst nightmare, or being overwhelmed with the intricate details of the number of micrograms of a specific nutrient within each meal – what I hope this book will give you is knowledge of the key foods to focus on throughout every stage of your life. Whether you're feeling great already and just want to do a little fine-tuning to ensure you're eating the right foods, or need help getting over health problems and want to know how you can enjoy eating the most nourishing foods in a practical and easy way, I hope Good Food for Life inspires you.

Keeping it simple

While searching for the words to introduce this, my eighth book, I came across two quotes which for me sum up why I've decided to write it – the first being the words of Voltaire.

'Nothing would be more tiresome than eating and drinking if God had not made them a pleasure as well as a necessity.'

Addressing the nutritional needs and appetites of every member of the family, each chapter follows a typical life stage – the prime years of adulthood, pregnancy and new life, feeding growing children, middle age, cooking for teenagers, and the over 60s. As such it will appeal to every woman with responsibilities, whether you are a mother, wife, lover, sister, daughter or friend. I've chosen not to focus on babies and toddlers as this is a specialised area that has been widely covered in much detail, not least in my own books Yummy! and Yummy Baby! Here I wanted to equip the woman typically at the heart of the family, whose stamina and dedication supports the wellbeing of a raft of others, right through midlife and beyond.

In the past I used to find a lot of enjoyment in spending a significant chunk of my time cooking, and I still do when I can manage to set aside a few hours at a weekend while my daughter Maya is out playing. But it's now more often the case that like most people, I'm juggling different aspects of my life: being a mum to the most gorgeous and smiley but minxy and chatty seven-year-old daughter, being alongside both my darling and my parents, and doing the work I love. My job involves a lot of travelling between the rural idyll where I write and my practices in London and Leicester and I find that balancing the different roles in the different locations requires me to simplify things far more than ever before.

Keeping things simple doesn't worry me; as you can see from books and films such as Food Inc and Fast Food Nation, there are worrying consequences in moving away from food that's as simply produced and locally sourced as we can get. I'm not a food-mile fanatic – we have to see far beyond food-mile labels and look at the overall environmental effect of both transportation and production in order to try and make an informed decision over whether a particular food is worth eating. I find all

Read more on:
◆ Pages
102–103 & 138

the equations so mind-boggling, that it's hard to decipher whether one food is more environmentally friendly to eat than another ◆ . So I have decided to pare down my decision-making process and my shopping habits, and working with the amazing Slow Food Movement (www.slowfood.org.uk), I do what I can to support good local food producers. It's easy to use the Internet to buy from passionate suppliers that I read and hear about from friends.

However, I'm not ashamed, and nor do I think anyone else should be, to buy produce from abroad – be this buffalo mozzarella from Puglia, prosciutto San Daniele, a slice of Brie or a German pumpernickel bread – for these should and can be part of our lives. I passionately believe we have great ingredients, food producers and chefs in our own countries, but we shouldn't think that we ought not to enjoy being part of a food world.

I also don't shy away from wanting to keep things simple when I'm cooking. People seem obsessed these days with trying to make a complicated meal every evening, especially for children, yet if we look back at the classic teas we grew up with – a lightly fried egg (or flat egg, as Maya calls it) on wholemeal toast or a bowl of pasta with a simple tomato sauce stirred through it – they are completely delicious and provide nourishment for a growing body (and an adult body who doesn't have the energy to make anything more complicated at the end of a long day).

As well as having basic cooking skills, we need to be able to work out the difference between true nutritional fact and the rubbish splashed across the newspaper headlines or in TV programmes. Pseudo-nutritionists' self-made nonsense has left a lot of people confused and feeling as if there's no way they can eat well and healthily in today's society. But nothing could be further from the truth – yes, it's hard with modern pressures to find the time to shop or know what's the best and most nourishing food to buy (not least when food companies are working hard to make their food look super-healthy with labels that aren't easy to decipher), but I hope you will find that you can actually glean all the nourishment you need from simple and delicious foods. For me, online delivery companies, which need not be expensive, are providing an incredibly important link between our farmers and small producers, and us, the consumers. Once you've sourced them and got into the routine of ordering, your goal of eating healthy and scrumptious food can be achieved; so let's keep my second quote, the words of Leonardo da Vinci, in the back of our minds.

'Simplicity is the ultimate sophistication.'

My favourite staples

I think we've lost our way a bit, being scared nowadays at seeing ingredients such as custard, cream, crème fraîche and butter in recipes, but it's perfectly possible to eat well and include these ingredients. In the recipe section (see pages 198–255) you'll find a selection of dishes that frequently appear on our table, and can be varied according to what's in season or what you fancy. All these recipes are good for the whole family, but in certain circumstances particular ones can be especially helpful, so I've given suggestions throughout the book to point you in the right direction.

If you're wondering about the calories, I hope this won't be a constant concern for you – it's not so much about how many calories foods have in them, it's whether these calories exist alongside anything nourishing in other ways. For example, a fig-stuffed Bramley apple with a dollop of Greek-style yoghurt will have more calories than the apple on its own, but as a breakfast, one of these will keep you satisfied until lunchtime. So really it's a question of how useful these calories are; if we look at the choice between, say, cooking with ingredients such as a nut butter as opposed to a low-fat spread, one will taste delicious and the other won't. And there is no difference between a large amount of a low-calorie food and a small delectable slice of something higher in calories – it's about controlling your appetite, savouring your food, cooking with good-quality ingredients and serving the food in a way that makes you feel satisfied in every sense.

I also feel with children that to ban sweet foods from the house is counterproductive and unnecessary; you build up the idea of a forbidden food being far more attractive, so they're likely to binge on it when you're not looking. If you cook some chocolate brownies using a good high-cocoa-bean chocolate, for example, the intensity of the chocolate is such that even the most chocolate-loving child will manage only a small piece. If you get them to enjoy it after a meal rather than on an empty stomach, the absorption of the sugar will be slower, which means it's less likely to send a sugar-sensitive child off in a tizzy. If you're trying to tempt the appetite of someone in their later years, a sliver of chocolate brownie with a drizzle of single cream will be sure to get them off the starting block.

Keeping a food diary

There are many occasions when it's helpful to keep a food diary. Often we don't realise what we're eating or how much of it, until it's written down in front of us. A carefully detailed record can be quite an eye-opener and may point to an obvious and simple solution.

It's also an extremely helpful record to take along if you need to seek medical advice. Try to include as much detail as possible and write down any changes and irregularities along with what you consider to be normal patterns.

DATE & TIME	FOOD & DRINK CONSUMED	QUANTITY	SYMPTOMS
	Give as much detail as you can about ingredients too. If your child is involved, they could collect and stick on the labels of anything they buy, such as confectionery, to make them feel part of the process and help you monitor their snacking away from home.	Use household measures, e.g. teaspoon, slice, small bowl etc.	Are you tired, constipated, nauseous? Do you have tummy aches or headaches? Has a rash appeared? Note down any changes to symptoms, which occur both before and after you've eaten.

Cooking and eating is serious business

I found it especially hard to keep within my allotted word count, particularly in the chapter on looking after teenagers, as there are some big issues to discuss. I think we're heading for huge problems with our next adult generation if we don't get food, cooking and eating in the home back on an even keel. The reason why so many young people struggle with obesity, eating disorders, anxiety over body image and mood swings – be this the usual typical teenage grumpiness and volatility or more serious depression – is that so many homes have become ready-meal reheating places rather than those where we sit together to eat and communicate. Often young girls start playing around with mad depleting diets and develop problems because there hasn't been enough good nourishing food in the house and no one has been able to take the time to teach them how to cook and eat properly. If you can keep some simple foods in the fridge and cupboard so that your teenagers can throw together something quick and nourishing, they'll be far less likely to want to go out for fast food. Yours will be the home their friends will want to come to eat at, and although this can be overwhelming at times, it gives you the opportunity watch what they're eating – you can pick up on eating-related problems, protect their bodies from being overwhelmed by too much fast food junk, and, above all, show love and affection through food and eating together.

When it comes to our later years, nourishing food becomes even more important, not least to meet the specific demands that an ageing body places on us but also to ensure that we are still fuelling our bodies with energy. This could be a body that's very fit and healthy, or one which has aged or is struggling with a health problem such as heart disease, dementia or cancer. As relatives and friends of older people, knowing which foods they can best nourish themselves with, and how to help them do this, provides an essential ingredient in living our lives alongside and caring for each other. So often hospitals and care homes get it wrong, as they seem to put the provision of delicious, nutritious food at the bottom of their list of priorities, so that even if you're healthy in old age, getting the right nourishment is difficult. For some older people, health problems arise for no other reason than the fact that they're not being catered for and looked after properly, which is scandalous and inexcusable. I just wait for the time when someone will sue their hospital or care home for the consequences of malnutrition; I can see the dangers of becoming litigious, but when it comes to a basic human right to be well fed and nourished, it's a cause worth fighting for.

Taking the time to enjoy a nutritious meal should be one of the most rewarding aspects of our later years. One of my favourite restaurants in Paris is Le Train Bleu, which is the most beautiful, ornate train restaurant at La Gare de Lyon. Elegant, mature Parisian women sit there in their finery, eating a small herb omelette accompanied by a green salad and a glass of wine. To me, this epitomises how elegant life and eating can be if we know what our bodies need, treasure the ingredients and know how to find and prepare them. Every stage of life can embrace this philosophy, and I look forward to moving on to the next phase knowing that I will still be able to enjoy food, and therefore, life.

Getting to grips with the boring science

I'm generally not a lover of charts and tables as I think we have become far too figure- and measure-focused. I prefer to think of meals like an Italian would – simple, delicious dishes, made up of handfuls of this and a dash of that – rather than obsessively looking at labels like a neurotic shopper. It's far easier as an adult to judge when you need more or less, but when feeding our children or elderly parents, it can sometimes be helpful to have a simple visual place to start. The eat well plate on the next page helps us see what food groups our bodies need. Actually, this is a model that applies to everyone over the age of five and can be gradually introduced for younger children, too as they begin to eat with the rest of the family.

You will see that the two biggest segments are carbohydrates and fibre and fruit and vegetables. Roughly one third of our intake should be from the first carbohydrate group of starches and one third from fruit and vegetables. Of the remaining third, most of it should be from the protein groups of milk and dairy, meat and fish, and non-dairy sources of protein such as tofu. Less than one sixth of our diet should be made up from the fat and sugar group, and of course it is best to eat good fats found in oily fish, nuts and seeds and more natural sugars, be this from fresh or puréed fruit or honey for sweetness. That said, cakes and puddings shouldn't be seen as an evil so long as they're eaten in the right proportions and ideally have some nourishing ingredients in them such as fruit, oats, wholemeal

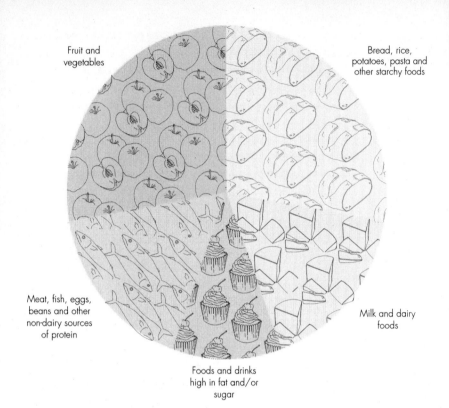

Fruit and vegetables

Bread, rice, potatoes, pasta and other starchy foods

Meat, fish, eggs, beans and other non-dairy sources of protein

Milk and dairy foods

Foods and drinks high in fat and/or sugar

Read more on: ◆ *Page 172*

flour, spelt ◆ , nuts, nut butters etc. Bear in mind that it isn't necessary to follow the model at every meal, but rather over a day or two.

Carbohydrates

Carbohydrates that are grain-based, as opposed to fruits and vegetables, are broken down into complex and simple varieties. These should form a large part of our diet because they are the best source of the energy you need in order to get around and to feel well and energetic. Complex carbs are incredibly rich in nutrients and give you consistent energy throughout the day, reducing the likelihood of you becoming tired and grumpy, which can be the case with simple refined carbohydrate/sugary foods.

The great complex carbs, which have had the least processing, are unsweetened mueslis, porridge oats, wholemeal and wholegrain breads, wholemeal muffins, pitta breads, cornbread, brown rice, millet, spelt, barley and buckwheat noodles. Simple carbohydrates are those that have had most of their fibre removed and may well have been bleached and refined – these are found in the white breads and pastas (and of course the biscuits and cakes) we see in the supermarket. We can usually, and indeed should try to, include some of these simple carbohydrates in our diet, unless as an adult you find that they just don't suit you. We should try not to make them our only source of carbohydrate because most of the goodness has been removed along with the husk of the grain, so we don't find as much of some of the minerals and vitamins that occur naturally in the complex carbohydrates. Most white flour used for bread is fortified with calcium ◆ , iron, niacin and other B vitamins, and this can be good especially for children and adults who aren't able to tolerate dairy products or simply don't like them. However, it's much better if you can include some wholemeal and wholewheat carbohydrates in your diet as well.

Read more on:
◆ Page 20
▲ Pages 66–67

Just as too much simple carbohydrate means we don't feel satisfied enough after eating (it's the fibre within the husk in complex carbs that makes you feel full), it's not good, especially for children and older people, to eat too many complex high-fibre carbs either. Too much wholegrain can be bulky and upset the gut, which means that you don't get enough energy from your food. As a result, young children (below 13 months) may not grow as well as they should, some people may feel tired all the time, and in extreme situations (though I've only seen this a few times) wholegrain can reduce the absorption of essential minerals such as iron and calcium. A lack of these minerals means children could develop weak bones and iron deficiency anaemia ▲, which though common in older people is thankfully rare in little ones.

Fibre

Fibre is needed to help keep our digestive system working efficiently and our hearts healthy; it also helps to balance our blood sugar, which affects our energy levels, our ability to concentrate and learn and reduces the chances of us developing conditions such as diabetes and certain cancers. Fibre is found in two main forms in our diets – soluble and insoluble – and we need both.

Soluble fibre is found mainly in fruits, vegetables, pulses and grains such as oats. Insoluble fibre is found in the husks of grains such as wheat and rye, so rye bread and the wholemeal varieties of bagels, muffins, cakes, etc. are rich sources. Insoluble fibre tends to keep the gut moving well and while soluble fibres can help the gut, they're more efficient in maintaining blood sugar levels and the heart through their positive effects on cholesterol and other fats in the blood. To maximise the amount of fibre in your diet, it's best to keep the peel on fruits such as apples and pears and to include some wholegrain products, such as porridge for breakfast or wholemeal bread in sandwiches.

Fruit and vegetables

Fruit and vegetables are also classified as complex carbohydrates and they're great for both children and adults. From the age of five you should be having five portions of fruit and veg a day, so that you get plenty of vitamins, minerals and fibre. Although we recommend five portions of fruit and vegetables a day, I think we'll soon be increasing this to seven, as there are so many benefits to eating a plentiful 'crop' of fruit and vegetables. Every cell in the body will benefit from the nutrients contained in fruits and vegetables.

It's good to vary the fruits and vegetables as much as possible because some are particularly rich in certain minerals and vitamins (spinach in iron and carrots in beta-carotene (vitamin A), for example). Tinned, frozen, cooked and dried fruits and vegetables can be as nutritious as fresh ones; if you bear in mind how practical they are, they can be great ingredients to turn to. If they've been heat-treated, tinned fruits and vegetables contain a little less vitamin C, but most manufacturers compensate for this by adding vitamin C to their products in supplement form. Opt for tinned fruits in natural fruit juice, not sugary syrup. Although wrongly seen as inferior, frozen fruits and vegetables are frozen soon after they have been picked, which means they are just as healthy as fresh (unless you're lucky enough to grow your own or have a generous neighbour, allotment or local market). I find frozen berries a particularly useful standby, and defrost them as and when I need them to use in smoothies, cereals, crumbles and compôtes. Fresh, raw fruits and vegetables usually contain more vitamins and minerals than cooked ones, but they can sometimes play havoc with your digestive system, in which case you may find that cooked fruits suit you better, for example: poached peaches or pears (in a juice such as orange juice, not in wine); baked apples; apricots, plums, greengages; or roasted and puréed vegetables such as roasted butternut squash with shavings of Pecorino cheese or pieces of buffalo mozzarella.

Proteins

Smoked haddock salad, page 224

Proteins are essential for growth, brain development, healthy bones and the production of happy hormones called endorphins. Amino acids are the building blocks of proteins and there are a total of 22 – eight of which (ten for children) are called essential because we can't make them in our body and must therefore get them from our food.

Proteins are divided into two groups: animal and plant. Animal proteins include chicken, seafood, fish, red or white meat from pork, beef, game and lamb, eggs, milk, butter, yoghurt and cheese. They are sometimes referred to as primary proteins, as they contain all eight essential amino acids and are considered to be the most important ones for growth. Plant foods rich in proteins are pulses, legumes, lentils, tofu and other soya products, and you can get some protein from cereal grains such as quinoa and from buckwheat and seaweed. As delicious as these foods are, they are referred to as incomplete proteins because they don't contain all of the essential amino acids, so you'll need to eat a combination of nuts, seeds and grains in order to receive all you need ♦. Children should have some protein along with carbohydrate every day, but adults don't always need the starch found in bread etc.

Read more on:
♦ Page 92

Roast mackerel with potatoes & thyme, page 215

Fats

We all, especially children and older people, need fats in our diet. Fats are necessary for brain function, particularly to help children learn, behave and concentrate; they provide some insulation under our skin so we don't lose too much body heat (this is particularly the case with older people); they produce essential hormones to ensure healthy growth and development, especially in children, teenagers and those wanting to become pregnant. Some fat is also needed to ensure good absorption of fat-soluble vitamins such as vitamin D.

The majority of normal-weight people should be eating enough good fat and not just tucking into low-fat foods, which can sometimes be high in sugar, taste inferior and leave you feeling deprived. It's all about knowing which are the better fats for us to eat. The long chain omega-rich fatty foods (see below) are most effective and good for virtually every part of the body. Other fats from dairy produce such as butter, cheese, cream, yoghurt and milk are fine to include in your diet, as in the right amount, they also contribute calcium, magnesium, vitamin A and a little vitamin D.

Omega-3 fatty acids

The most effective omega-3 fats occur naturally in oily fish as eicosapentaenoic acid (EPA) and docosahexaenoic acid (DHA). They also occur naturally in seeds as alpha-linolenic acid (ALA). Good sources include linseed (flaxseed) oil, linseeds, soya bean oil, pumpkin seeds, walnut oil, rapeseed oil and soya beans. They are good for healthy brain function, the heart, joints, and general wellbeing.

The body can convert ALA into EPA and DHA, but not very efficiently. This is why oily fish plays such an important role in a non-vegetarian diet. Oily fish contain EPA and DHA in a ready-made form, which enables the body to use it easily. The main sources of oily fish include salmon, trout, mackerel, herring, sardines, pilchards and kippers, either fresh, frozen, canned or smoked. Unfortunately the exception is tinned tuna, as it doesn't contain the high levels of omega oils found in fresh and frozen tuna but is still a good source of protein.

Vitamins and minerals

The reason I haven't included a specific nutrients chart, with quantities of this and that, is that I want you to feel completely free to find out what works for your own body. Everyone is different and our needs change constantly – one day we may need to stock up on a plentiful supply of energy, while other days we rely on these stores to keep us going. Both of these scenarios are fine, but it's important to know the sort of nutritious food pillars you should try to include each day, bearing in mind that on days when you're not able to nourish your body as well as you'd like, your body will have enough in reserve. There are plenty of websites and books that will give you more detail in milligrams and micrograms, charts and diagrams, but I want Good Food for Life to be the place you turn to for inspiration, just as much as knowledge.

Fat-soluble vitamins

Vitamins are classified as fat- or water-soluble. Fat-soluble vitamins are absorbed with fat through the intestine into the circulation and then stored in the liver.

Vitamin A (beta-carotene) is needed for healthy growth, skin, teeth and vision. It protects against infections and is a powerful antioxidant, so helps prevent diseases such as heart disease and cancer. The best sources are cantaloupe melon, pumpkin, squash, carrots, peaches, apricots, red and orange peppers, tomatoes, liver, egg yolk, dairy produce, mackerel and herrings.

Vitamin D is important for the absorption of calcium, building and maintaining strong, healthy bones and teeth. It also helps muscle function and works with vitamins A and C to boost your immune system. Vitamin D is mainly manufactured by the skin when it's exposed to sunlight, but the following foods are also good sources: sardines, herrings, salmon, tuna, dairy produce and eggs.

Vitamin E is an antioxidant needed for healthy skin, a good strong immune system, a healthy heart, and in creams helps reduce scarring. It's found in all vegetable oils, avocados, broccoli, almonds, sunflower seeds, eggs, soya and wholegrains, which include oatmeal, rye and brown rice.

Vitamin K is great for building and maintaining healthy, strong bones and essential for helping blood to clot properly – you may recall that babies are given an injection of vitamin K straight after birth. Vitamin K can be found in bio yoghurt, egg yolks, fish oils, dairy produce and green leafy vegetables.

Water-soluble vitamins

With the exception of vitamin B12, which is stored in the liver, water-soluble vitamins remain in the body for a short time before being excreted by the kidneys – so you need to keep up your intake.

Vitamin B1 is needed for energy production, carbohydrate digestion, heart function and helps children concentrate and their brains generally to function well. It is found in wholegrain foods, such as good cereals and bread, oats, rye, millet, quinoa, legumes, pork and liver.

Vitamin B2 is needed for digestion of carbohydrates, but also fats and proteins, and generally helps our bodies derive enough energy from food. It's also needed for hair, nails and the development of sex organs. The best sources are bio yoghurt, fish, liver, milk, cottage cheese and green leafy vegetables such as spinach.

Vitamin B3 (also known as niacin) is good for the sex hormones and other hormones connected to the digestive system, such as insulin, the hormone that regulates blood sugar levels in the body, and also for thyroxine, serotonin and other mood and brain hormones. Vitamin B3 is generally found in the same foods as vitamins B1 and B2.

Vitamin B5 is needed for conversion of fats and carbohydrates into energy and also for supporting the adrenal glands, which regulate the stress response in the body. It also ensures a strong immune system. We find it in wholegrains, rye, barley, millet, nuts, chicken, egg yolks, liver and green leafy vegetables.

Vitamin B6 is needed for a strong nervous system, for an equally robust immune system and to help repair the body when it gets injured. The main sources include poultry such as chicken and turkey, lean red meat, egg yolks, oily fish, dairy produce, cabbage, leeks and wheat germ.

Folic acid or folate, if from the natural source (vitamin B9) is perhaps most famous for its role in preventing neural defects during pregnancy, but it's also good for the immune system, energy production and preventing anaemia ◆. It's found in good old dark green leafy vegetables such as kale, spinach, asparagus, broccoli, Brussels sprouts, egg yolks, carrots, apricots, oranges and orange juice, pumpkins and squashes, melons (particularly the cantaloupe variety), wholewheat and rye. You can also get cereals and bread fortified with synthetic folic acid.

Read more on: ◆ *Pages 66–67*

Vitamin B12 is needed for growth, digestion and nerves, as well as the production of energy and healthy blood cells. It's found in red meats such as beef, liver and pork, shellfish and other fish, eggs and dairy produce; for vegetarians, you can also find it in seaweed and spirulina.

Vitamin C is needed for a strong immune system, a healthy heart, good skin, preventing diseases like heart disease and cancer in later life, and helping bumps, scratches and cuts to heal properly. The best sources are kiwi fruits, blueberries (in fact, all berries), pomegranates, citrus fruits, potatoes, pumpkins and squashes, sweet peppers, green leafy vegetables, cabbage, broccoli, cauliflower and spinach.

Biotin is needed for hair and nails, skin and energy production. It's found in brewer's yeast, brown rice, nuts, egg yolks and fruit.

Minerals

Calcium is essential for bones, teeth and the heart, and is needed to help our muscles work properly. It's found in dairy produce, small-boned fish such as sardines and anchovies, green leafy vegetables (except spinach, which contains oxalic acid, hindering our ability to absorb calcium), soya products such as soya milk, soya mince and tofu, almonds, sesame seeds (so tahini and hummus are great), sunflower seeds (which I roast and give Maya as a snack with sultanas and raisins) and dried fruits such as apricots. You can also buy calcium-fortified breads, even orange juice, although it's much better to get most of your calcium requirement from natural sources.

As dairy products are a rich source of calcium, three portions each day should be sufficient to meet an adult's daily need of 700mg of calcium. Choose low or reduced fat versions to avoid too much unhealthy saturated fat. A portion includes a glass (200ml/scant cup) of full-fat (whole), semi-skimmed, 1 per cent or skimmed milk; 250ml (1 cup) calcium-fortified soya milk; 40g (1½oz) cheese, such as Cheddar, Brie, feta, mozzarella or Stilton; 125g (4½oz) soft cheese, such as cottage cheese or fromage frais; a small pot (150g/⅔ cup) of low-fat plain or fruit yoghurt; fruit smoothie made with 200ml (scant cup) milk or 150g (⅔ cup) yoghurt.

Iron is important for growth and development and crucial in the production of healthy red blood cells, which carry oxygen around the body. It can be found in liver, lean red meat and egg yolks, as well as foods suitable for vegetarians such as lentils, fortified breakfast cereals, dried apricots and figs, nuts, spinach, kale, seaweed (if you can get your children to eat it!), watercress, broccoli, baked beans, oatmeal, avocados, asparagus, sunflower and sesame seeds and fresh herbs, particularly parsley.

Magnesium helps the body deal with stress, generate enough energy and build strong healthy bones. It also helps the muscle and nervous systems. It's found in citrus fruits, green vegetables such as broccoli, cabbage, nuts and seeds, bread, fish, meat, dairy produce, dried fruits (especially figs and raisins), tomatoes, garlic, carrots, potatoes, aubergines, onions and sweetcorn.

Selenium, which works alongside other antioxidants such as vitamin E, is essential for the immune system and to protect us from skin cancer. It's found in brazil nuts, which can be ground into a delicious mix with seeds to sprinkle on cereals or in porridge, all fresh fruits and vegetables, shellfish, sesame seeds, wheat germ and bran (so healthy cereals are a good source), tomatoes and broccoli.

Zinc is best known for being involved in the immune system, but it's also good for sexual development, regulating moods, the nervous system and brain function. Sources include fish and shellfish, lean red meats, wholegrains, poultry, nuts and seeds, eggs, cauliflower, berries, dairy produce such as yoghurt, oats, rye, wheat germ, brown rice and buckwheat.

Potassium is found abundantly in many foods, and is especially easy to obtain in fruits and vegetables such as chard, mushrooms, and spinach. It can help your muscles and nerves to function properly, lower your risk of high blood pressure and heart problems, ease fatigue, irritability and confusion, and reduce chronic diarrhoea. Older people are more at risk of too much potassium in the body as their kidneys are less able to eliminate any excess.

Sodium is a component of salt, which is naturally present in the majority of foods. Most people eat more salt than is good for their health. It's recommended that adults eat no more than 6g of salt (equivalent to 2.5g of sodium per day). The daily recommendations for children are 2g (1–3 years old), 3g (4–6 years old), 5g (7–10 years old) and 6g (11+ years old). Three-quarters of our salt consumption comes from packaged foods, such as breakfast cereals, soups, sauces and ready meals, so it's easy to inadvertently have too much. Don't mistake sodium levels on labels for the salt content – you need to multiply this by 2.5 to get the salt value ◆.

Read more on: ◆ Page 44

Food storage

Something I've found that makes an enormous difference to how fresh and tasty food stays is to look closely at how we wrap and store it. For example, transferring opened tinned foods into sealed plastic containers stops the food being spoilt by contact with the air and metal – once you lose the protective heat-treated seal of the unopened tin, food can spoil very quickly. Often re-sealing technology doesn't live up to expectations, and you're better off taking the food out of the packet and putting it into a plastic container or a good-quality resealable bag. With good wrapping, we not only reduce our risk of food poisoning, but also reduce our food wastage and the contribution that makes to carbon emissions from landfill sites.

If you haven't already found them, try the specially designed food-preserving bags that can make a bag of salad leaves last for days after opening instead of collapsing and drying up. Banana bags, indulgent as they sound, keep bananas fresh as you can store them in the fridge for a couple of weeks (without these special bags bananas go black in the fridge).

Making the most of your fridge

Try not to put too much food into your fridge, as you want the air to circulate properly – this keeps the temperatures at the required levels to keep the food fresh and not spoil. As with cupboards, stock them in rotation so that you use the older yoghurts, etc. before new ones.

Most butchers don't recommend leaving uncooked meat or poultry wrapped in clingfilm or plastic for long, as it goes slimy and can't breathe. Ideally, remove all packaging and wrap it in greaseproof paper, then put it on a plate so that it doesn't drip anywhere. Cold cuts and salamis dry out easily, so wrap them well. Fresh and smoked fish can stay in its sealed bag and is best well wrapped.

Cheese tends to sweat and spoil more easily wrapped in clingfilm – it keeps better in waxed paper, which prevents it from drying out. Oils and butters can go rancid with heat and time (oxidised fats are unstable and aren't good for the heart), so buy enough butter for the week or freeze it in small portions. I'm careful to keep bottles of oil in a cool place away from the cooker, and I keep special extra virgin oils in the fridge (they turn cloudy as they cool, so you need to get them out about an hour before you want to use them). Eggs are often debated over – I don't keep mine in the fridge, but many recommend you do, as this maximises freshness. However, cold eggs tend to crack more easily when you boil them, and if you want to make meringues or mayonnaise you need to get them out of the fridge for a few hours beforehand.

Fruit and vegetables are best left unwashed before they're popped into the fridge, but I tend to wash everything apart from salad and soft berry fruits (best left in their punnets) beforehand, as it means I can just grab something as I fly out of the door. Do check out the stay-fresh-longer bags as they've made a real difference to my food spend and to how much enjoyment Maya gets out of a crisp, fresh-tasting carrot as opposed to a slightly off-peak one. It's always a good idea to wash salad in fresh, cold water and eat it within a day of purchasing. Pure fruit and no-added-sugar jams need to be stored in the fridge, as they don't have the usual high sugar content to act as a preservative.

Be aware of food poisoning

Don't panic if your child picks up a bit of food off your kitchen floor and pops it into their mouth – it's not ideal, but it won't kill them and there are real advantages for their immune systems if you don't keep them in a sterile environment. Children (and adults) need to get into the habit of washing their hands after going to the toilet and before meals, but at the same time, the old saying 'Dirt is good' is true. However, when cooking for young children and older people, you need to be vigilant with food hygiene because they are more at risk of poisoning from wrongly stored or badly cooked food. Food poisoning is more common when budgets are stretched, as it can be tempting to think that best-before dates can be extended a little to help eke out the shop for a few more days. Although with correct storage some extra time can be safe, as with food hygiene, you need to be careful when it comes to children, older people or anyone with a compromised or vulnerable immune system. Best-before dates are there for a reason – to protect us from food poisoning bacteria – so take notice of them even if it means wasting food.

The freezer – my life saver

Now I'm a mum, I'd be lost without my freezer. Not only does it mean that I can cook meals in advance, but also, from a very practical point of view, it has simplified my shopping routine. I tend to freeze portions of sausages and bread, and also freeze milk (which has to be pasteurised). I also freeze small bags of freshly grated Parmesan, as the taste is far superior to the ready-grated kind. Eggs can be frozen if they're beaten lightly (don't freeze whole), either yolk and white together or separated into yolks and whites for use in sauces or to make meringues. You can freeze egg whites without doing anything to them, but with yolks you need to beat them a little and add a pinch of salt or sugar (remember to label which you've added!). Boiled eggs, mayonnaise, custard, yoghurt (unless it's made into a frozen yoghurt pudding) and single cream don't freeze well, although double cream can be frozen when whipped.

Don't use frozen food for dishes that require re-freezing, as not only can this affect the texture of the dish, but more importantly it may increase the risk of food spoilage or poisoning bugs growing. Freezing doesn't kill all bacteria, which is why you must make sure all food is well wrapped in special freezer bags, plastic containers or extra strong foil, and that it is reheated and defrosted thoroughly. Remember that young children and older people are more likely to get ill with food poisoning, so you need to be extra careful that you reheat to the correct temperatures to completely cook the food. It's fine to then let it cool down a little, but make sure you don't just heat it to a lukewarm temperature you think is right for your little one to eat, as if you do this not all the bugs will have been killed.

Freezing is also a good way to take advantage of good buys in supermarkets, as you can buy more for less money and most importantly not waste any. Picking your own fruit and popping it into the freezer is best of all, as you're getting the most nutritious fruit fresh from the plant. For a family a freezer is a life and sanity saver, and the frozen produce can be great nutritionally as well as in cost value.

Freezing bread

Bread freezes well but goes stale more easily in the fridge, so to make best use of a loaf, divide it as soon as you've brought it and freeze it in manageable quantities – if you're making a packed lunch it works well to freeze a couple of slices in a small bag and take it out of the freezer last thing at night. It also means you can have different breads on different days and not have to waste any. If bread is more than a few days old turn it into croutons or use it for bread and butter pudding or as the base of a soup. It can also be whizzed up to make breadcrumbs (which can also be frozen) to use as a coating for fish fingers or chicken drumsticks, or to go in burgers, falafels, home-made sausages or stuffing.

Freezing fruit

Most fruits freeze well, and this can also be a good way to preserve some vitamin C. Freezing puts a time freeze on the natural reduction in vitamin C, meaning you end up with fruits higher in vitamin C once they come out of the freezer.

Berry fruits are best frozen separately on trays, then packed together in plastic containers. Stone fruits such as plums, damsons and peaches can be frozen with stones in, but I tend to take the stones out and then, like berries, freeze them separately on trays and pack them together once frozen. They're all great for future jam, fruit sauce, chutney and compôte making. With cooked fruits I've got into the habit of filling small freezer bags that I can take out and throw into the microwave for a few minutes if I want a late afternoon snack or in the mornings for Maya to have with porridge (it takes only about five minutes to go from frozen to hot).

Citrus fruits freeze surprisingly well – simply peel and segment oranges (ideally seedless) and freeze as above to make delicious little popsicles for children. This is also a good base for making marmalade if you have a glut of oranges, lemons, limes, grapefruits or other citrus fruit. Finely grated lemon, lime and orange rinds freeze well in ice-cube trays and are great for adding to fruit crumbles, cakes, curries, etc.

Freezing herbs and spices

Herbs and spices can be made economical and practical to grow by freezing them, chopped, in ice-cube trays, to be popped out ready to season sauces, tagines, curries, casseroles, soups, etc. I don't think frozen herbs work as well in raw dishes, as they're slightly mushy when thawed. Alternatively make up a batch of herb-based sauces, such as basil pesto. I find that grated fresh ginger also freezes well and is a great addition to soups, stir-fries and curries.

The natural oiliness of spices means that they can turn rancid easily in a hot light kitchen, leaving the final dish somewhat fusty and unpleasant. So only buy small amounts at a time and ideally store them in small dark jars and in a cool place. Whole spices tend to last longer and give a fresher taste. You can freeze most spices as long as they are well wrapped.

Check out your cupboards

Like the fridge and freezer, if you look at the way you store dry and tinned foods, the family shop will stretch further and the food will stay fresh, taste good and reduce the likelihood of any little creatures making a nest! The ideal is a cool, dark larder with slate or tiled shelves and racks for vegetables, etc., but this isn't usually the norm. The best choice of cupboard in which to store your food should be as cool as possible, not near an oven, and well ventilated. Even tinned and packet foods will deteriorate and spoil in hot rooms.

Dried goods such as flour can grow moulds – especially the wholewheat versions, which contain more fat because the grains have natural oils in them. Storage jars are ideal for opened dry goods, but remember not to just top them up but use the oldest rice, pasta, etc. first. Tear off the use-by date from the packet and pop it into the jar so that you can keep on top of using food at its best. Cereals can go off and lose their freshness quicker than you think, so keep the waxed inside packets tightly sealed or transfer into storage jars if little hands have loosened their packaging. The same applies to porridge oats – there is a natural oiliness in the whole flakes of oats, so keep them well wrapped. As tempting as BOGOF (buy one get one free) deals are, they often make us buy too much food, so that you end up eating it past its best or throwing it away – unless you're a dab hand with the freezer, in which case making a big batch of pasta sauce with tomatoes bought on offer is ideal.

In Your Prime

Having endured the teenage years and come out the other side relatively unscathed, our bodies now enter the prime age. Generally considered as our 20s, 30s and 40s, we should be looking and feeling our strongest and best. In theory, being an adult brings autonomy but in practice we are hit by all sorts of demands. Finding time to shop for the sorts of nourishing foods you know you should be eating and having the energy to cook alongside the pressures of everyday life, isn't easy for anyone, including me.

But what I'm hoping you'll gather from this book is that there is nothing wrong with the occasional day or meal when there isn't a salad, fruit or wholegrain in sight – for me a classic comfort meal would be delicious sourdough bread, thinly sliced and toasted, along with a board of cheeses and a good tangy pickle – and also that nourishing foods can be quick and easy to prepare as long as you have well-stocked cupboards. This can help you to live healthily and yet still lead a rewarding work and social life – not the easiest of balances to get right.

As to what your body needs now that you've moved into a life stage that doesn't involve as much growth and development as when you were a young child or a teenager, the foundations are in essence the same as for any other stage in life – you need a balance of different nourishing foods to enable you to feel and look your best.

Our body needs fuel

How much food we need largely depends on what sort of day we have ahead of us and how our body is feeling. On average we say that three meals a day with a couple of nutritious snacks in between is a good pattern to work to. However, whenever the work and home environments produce practical and emotional challenges, we can be fooled into thinking that because we feel hungry and may not have time for a proper lunch, it's okay to grab some nibbles or reward a stressful afternoon by dipping into a stash of chocolate biscuits.

Don't forget that the body often craves the distraction of eating – you start to feel hungry when really you want an excuse to take a break or need some classic oral satisfaction – yes, food can be a comfort, but not when it ruins your appetite for a nourishing breakfast, lunch or evening meal. You may feel that working long hours requires you to eat more, especially if you feel hungry, but the reality is that unless you're involved in an extremely active job or working out big-time in the gym, if you answer every hunger pang with a nibble, your weight is quickly going to start piling on.

If it's a break you need, have a drink of something that's not loaded in sugar and fats – it's no surprise, I'm sure, to hear me say that a can of a fizzy, sugary drink can tot up an astronomical sugar hit that shouldn't be ignored. A can of cola can contain as much sugar as a slice of delicious, gooey chocolate cake, although admittedly without the fat (but I'd rather have the chocolate cake!). Don't be misled into thinking that a glass of fruit juice doesn't deliver a sugar hit of its own, because it does, in the form of fructose. Fructose in its original form within a piece of fresh fruit, should be considered as a different thing from when it is drunk as a juice or smoothie. Although juice contains useful vitamins and minerals, the fructose can cause just as much of a sugar high feeling, and therefore a sugar crash, as an artificially flavoured canned drink. It has the same hefty calorie hit, which can really start to add up if you're a big fruit juice drinker. When it comes to your teeth, the stickiness of thicker fruit juices such as smoothies, while delicious, can hang around in the mouth more than a thin juice and corrode teeth. Apart from the sugar content which causes decay, too many fruit drinks can erode enamel and stain teeth.

Watch the energy-rich foods

You may have been one of those teenagers who could eat almost anything they liked – fry-ups, takeaways, snacks of chocolate mid-afternoon – without affecting your weight, but when we reach our mid-20s and go through to our 40s, the chances are that our metabolism will slow down and the effects on our health begin to show. Unless we're careful either with the quantities of fats and sugars we consume or are very active, our weight will go in the wrong direction – up and out. Even if our weight doesn't change, our body shape can – more fat can accumulate around the bits we often have hang-ups about, such as hips, waist, etc., so we start to feel negative about our body. On the inside, excess saturated fat in particular can cause a rise in levels of the bad sort of cholesterol (LDL – see below), which can cause all sorts of health problems. Diets rich in saturated fatty acids are also associated with the development of insulin resistance, which can contribute to developing diabetes ◆, and dyslipidaemia (abnormal blood fat levels) as part of 'Metabolic Syndrome' (a cluster of risk factors for cardiovascular disease).

Read more on:
◆ *Page 149*

HDL and LDL cholesterol

There are two types of cholesterol: high-density lipoprotein (HDL), or 'good', and low-density lipoprotein (LDL), or 'bad'. LDL is the kind of cholesterol that can be deposited in our arteries and cause problems, while HDL is the good kind, which picks up LDL and takes it back to the liver to be broken down. HDL helps to counteract the damaging effects of LDL – so, put perhaps more simply, we should keep our LDL levels down and try to boost HDL. Below 5mmol/l (millimoles per litre) (193mg/dl) is our preferred total cholesterol level, but to make up this figure the ideal is that LDL cholesterol should be 3.0mmol/l (116 mg/dl) or less and HDL cholesterol should be 1.2mmol/l (46 mg/dl) or more. The TC/HDL ratio (that is, your total cholesterol divided by your HDL cholesterol) should be 4.5 or less. This reflects the fact that for any given total cholesterol level, the more HDL the better. It's the balance between these two types of cholesterol that (along with eliminating other risk factors such as smoking, diabetes and high blood pressure) really protects us against the risk of heart disease and stroke.

This means watching foods rich in saturated fats – butter, cream, cheese, fatty meats and foods containing all of these ingredients – as once inside the body, the liver turns this fat into cholesterol.

Cholesterol-busting tips

- Use skimmed (fat-free), semi-skimmed or 1 per cent milk (slightly lower than semi-skimmed) and look to the cheeses that are lower in fat or eat less of the full-fat cheeses.
- Choose lean cuts of meat such as steaks, or good-quality, high-meat-content sausages. Another tip is to buy good-quality, low-fat sausage meat, mix it with falafel-type ingredients such as chickpeas, herbs and spices, roll it into balls and cook them like little rissoles. Alternatively make a sausage, tomato and potato pie and serve with ratatouille, caponade or roasted vegetables.
- Cuts of meat such as brisket, oxtail, ham hocks and shoulders and braising steak, are economical to buy. These can usually benefit from longer, slower cooking methods such as casseroling,

making hot pots or tagines, and the meat can be made more tender by marinating. It's a good idea to cook these dishes the day before, so you remove the excess fat that forms on the surface when left to cool, but so often the flavours improve with time and through reheating.

- Don't be put off by cheaper cuts of meat that have some fat marbled through them – the cooking process requires some fat for flavour and tenderness, and overly lean meat can be as tough as old boots. Use a good-quality, not over-fatty meat and remove the excess fat after cooking. You can buy fat-removing brushes or use kitchen paper to soak up any excess fat. Using a non-stick frying pan helps, as does using a minimal amount of oil.

Focus on fibre

Read more on:
◆ Pages 18–21
▲ Pages 171–172

Chicken & chickpea burgers, page 212

Fibre is one of our best allies. When we're young, too many fibre-rich foods can fill us up, preventing our body from gleaning enough energy from our diet and absorbing key minerals ◆. When we become adults, the benefits of having a diet rich in fibrous foods are so great, and the downsides are usually so minimal – exceptions arise for people with a sensitive digestion, such as those with IBS ▲ – that we can simply say for the majority of us that the more fibre we can eat the better. But that doesn't mean we can plough our way through a loaf of wholemeal bread, as this will tot up many calories and leave our stomach feeling completely stuffed. What I mean is that if we can look at the foods we eat and see if we can incorporate a higher-fibre version, or add some fibre-rich foods to a meal, this will most likely bring some tangible benefits.

The advantage of boosting the amount of fibre in our diet is that within hours, if not sooner, we will start to feel different. Okay, to begin with when we start eating more fibre we might feel a little bloated, but this is normal and due to the fact that we've changed our diet and it takes a while for the gut to adjust and feel great. (By the way, we should always ensure that we drink plenty of water when we boost our fibre, as this helps the fibre to work and prevents constipation – surprisingly, even though fibre is usually good for preventing this, in the short term fibre and no water can bung us up.) Eating fibre-rich foods correctly can help alleviate bloating, constipation and provide other short- and long-term benefits.

You might think the fibre message is one that is well and truly understood, but in fact we're just not eating enough of it. We should be eating 18g (¾ oz) a day, yet the average for an adult is only 12g (½ oz) – which, bearing in mind that this is the average, means there are many people falling way below the 18g (¾ oz) a day target. This is why so many people have digestive problems, don't feel satiated enough after their meals and are therefore more inclined to overeat and be overweight.

Here's a little science. The term 'fibre' is branded around on products and in marketing messages but it sometimes isn't as well understood as it should be. The connotation of 'fibre' is that it tends to equate with boring and worthy foods, when really it could perhaps benefit from a touch of re-branding so that people would associate it with satisfaction. It's wondrously beneficial in so many ways and at the same time it can be delicious. The word actually describes something we used to call 'roughage', which doesn't sound very pleasant in my book, but in a way this describes it better, as fibre consists of the edible parts of plants that are not broken down and absorbed in our small intestine.

You may have seen the terms 'soluble' and 'insoluble' bandied around, and in essence these are different types of fibre which are named according to the kind of beneficial effect they have in our body. Some (insoluble) are better at helping to get the gut moving as it should, and therefore are the ones to focus on when you're trying to prevent constipation, while others (soluble) are better at helping us to control blood cholesterol and the sugar levels in our blood – which can then have an impact on our energy levels, the temptation to nibble and moods. The reason you should try to incorporate a good mix of soluble and insoluble fibre is in order to glean the benefits right across the board – from reducing bowel problems right the way through to feeling satiated when you've eaten, having healthy blood fat and well-controlled blood sugar levels.

The different types of fibre in the foods we eat behave differently when they meet the bacteria that lives in our large intestine – some fibrous foods are partly fermented, others completely, by these gut bacteria, and this fermentation process, unpleasant as it sounds, is something we want to encourage. This is because the gases produced, such as carbon dioxide, methane and hydrogen, and short-chain fatty acids (butyrate, acetate and propionate), are extremely beneficial to our health. For instance, the short-chain fatty acids are absorbed into the cells of the gut wall, where they can be used as fuel, or pass on into the bloodstream, where they can have all sorts of positive effects such as decreasing the risk of developing bowel cancer ◆. This is one of the most common cancers alongside breast and lung cancer, and hundreds of people are diagnosed with the disease every day. Eating a diet rich in fibre is one of the most effective ways to prevent the disease.

Read more on:
◆ Pages 128–131
▲ Page 20

Chickpea, tomato & sausage hot pot, page 202

Essential iron

Iron is an important nutrient for growth and development ▲ but something that many people (women in particular) tend to lack. One of the reasons for this is that we used to be much bigger red meat eaters than we are these days – maybe it's fears over the relationship between poor-quality, fatty red meat and the development of heart disease and cancer, or the fact that for moral reasons we are preferring to eat more of a fish, white meat or vegetarian diet. I don't eat as much red meat as I used to simply because I prefer to eat more of everything else – I love bean- and lentil-based dishes such as dahl or curry, or a chickpea tabouleh-style salad with roasted vegetables, more than a simple roast – and I admit I'm fussy about where I source my meat, so would rather wait until I can get hold of meat that I have confidence in eating. I also try to make red meat go further – I'd prefer to pay a little more for good-quality, well-sourced brisket of beef and make it stretch to a couple of meals: first making a casserole slow-cooked with root vegetables, then mincing up the cooked meat to make a shepherd's pie, and often making a third meal by using the vegetables and meat as a soup.

Sometimes, however, I crave a good steak, most often on a Friday evening when I'm tired, and this is completely healthy. Most of the studies that link red meat with ill health either don't distinguish whether we're talking about a fatty red meat product such as low-meat-content high-fat sausages, or a lean good-quality steak – and there is a vast difference. It's perfectly possible to be healthy and eat meat if you ensure that it isn't high in fat and that your overall diet is rich enough in other nutritious foods to ensure that your blood fat levels (one of the chief concerns over a diet heavy in fatty red meat) stay within the ideal range. I would say that eating good-quality red meat once or twice a week is about the right frequency.

If meat turns your stomach and you need to up your iron intake, there are non-meat sources of iron such as dark green leafy vegetables, eggs, soya, dried fruits like prunes, figs and apricots, fortified breakfast cereals, etc., but the iron is not as well absorbed by the body. You need to ensure that in the same meal you have some food that's rich in vitamin C, as this will help your body absorb the iron ◆. In practical terms this could mean either a fresh fruit salad or bowl of fresh berries after a meal or a glass of freshly squeezed juice. Bear in mind that frozen vegetables can contain more vitamin C than so-called fresh, which can make the practical issues of boosting fresh veg and fruit in the diet easier.

Read more on:
◆ Page 20
▲ Pages 35–36
● Pages 36–38

Oxtail soup, page 232

Be careful not to reduce iron absorption

Check that you're not having too much tannin in tea, as this inhibits the absorption of iron – tannins are not to be confused with caffeine, as they're two completely different things, and decaffeinated teas contain just as much tannin as normal tea. One option is to go for herbal teas ▲; alternatively you don't need to refrain from enjoying a proper 'cuppa', but instead of having it with or straight after a meal, leave it a couple of hours so that the tannins within the tea don't interfere with the iron absorption. Tannin levels within a cup of tea increase the longer you leave the leaves seeping, so a lighter-coloured, weaker tea is another way to reduce tannin levels. This brings caffeine levels down as well – although caffeine doesn't have as negative an effect on iron absorption as tannins – but you do need to watch that you don't take in too much caffeine for your general health ●.

Phytates in bran and oxalates in spinach, nuts, chocolate, parsley and rhubarb can reduce the iron effect too, so just make sure you're choosing other green leafy vegetables as well as spinach and that your diet isn't too bran-based.

A warming cup of tea

The average Briton consumes a phenomenal 2.5kg (5½ lb) of tea a year, second only to the Irish globally, while ironically in India and China, where some of the finest teas are grown, the annual consumption is more like 500g (18oz). There is a lot to be said in favour of tea, not least what a delicious restorative beverage it can be. Drinking tea, whether black, white, green, or something more exotic-sounding like Oolong or rooibos, is now seen as a good way to take in antioxidants and other substances known as bioactives that may help reduce the incidence not only of heart disease, but also of Alzheimer's and other types of dementia ◆.

Read more on:
◆ Pages 189 & 195–197
▲ Page 20

Drinking a cup of tea is a great way to top up your fluid intake. Although I'm a huge fan of water and there is a slight diuretic effect in tea, so that we don't glean quite as much water as we would from hot water and lemon, sometimes a cup of tea just hits the spot. It can be an easy and enticing way to take in the benefits of milk, such as calcium ▲, and a little caffeine. It's less potent a caffeine hit than coffee would be, and it may suit you not to have as powerful an energiser – I can drink tea when I'm anxious and it will be calmative, whereas a coffee would tip me into feeling more jittery and anxious.

Herbal teas are not only a great alternative to black, white, green etc., but also have many useful medicinal properties. I don't see the harm in looking to traditional herbal teas, as we could do well to just listen to our ancestors; just ask your doctor or pharmacist if you're taking medication of any sort – most of the ingredients in herbal teas are safe, but herbs are drugs and therefore can be as potent as some medications, particularly when drunk in large quantities. We're quite right to be more careful with children and not to let them drink too much of it, but if they're well, there is nothing wrong with them having a cup of tea. It's warming, soothing, and far better for them than a fizzy drink.

Although research is still in its infancy in terms of real-life tea drinkers (as opposed to a laboratory result), we are able to deduce that the antioxidants found in teas in varying amounts may well be useful in fighting the day-to-day battle of preventing heart disease, and these antioxidants, along with substances we call bioactives, may have a role to play in keeping our brains healthy and our immune systems strong.

Quality is everything

One of the frustrations I have when choosing tea in some supermarkets is that it's very hard to find out much about it, other than assuming that the more you pay for it the finer the quality (though this isn't always the case). For this reason I like to support and source passionate small tea producers, who source the teas themselves and can give you so much information about individual varieties. I particularly like silver tip tea, which is unique in that it is just the leaf buds that are used, unlike all other teas, which are made up of the opened leaves. These mature buds have not yet opened to the sun and therefore have not begun to photosynthesise, making them especially low in caffeine and tannins.

White, green, Oolong and black teas all come from the leaves of Camellia sinensis. White and green tea are set apart by the way they are processed. Black teas are processed through fermentation, which results in some of the beneficial nutrients being converted into other compounds. Green tea, however, is steamed to prevent oxidisation and retains more antioxidants, which have been attributed to making it more effective at preventing and fighting various diseases. White tea is the least processed of all teas and therefore contains the highest concentrates of antioxidants. In the Far East, white silver tip tea has long been used as an aphrodisiac and is known for its ability to soothe a hangover. Oolong is a tea that falls between black and green tea and undergoes only a small amount of fermentation during processing. Some laboratory studies have suggested that it is good for enhancing the body's ability to metabolise fats, largely because of its extremely high levels of a particular bioactive called polyphenol, but we're far from being able to say that this would be able to have an impact on global obesity and heart disease. But watch this research!

Water is best fresh and should not be re-boiled, since the oxygen content is diminished, which affects the tea. For black, green and white tea the water should be below boiling point because the amino acids (which produce the tea's flavour) dissolve at lower temperatures than tannin. Tea made with water at 100°C will be more astringent and less sweet. Ideally you should stop the kettle when small bubbles form along the sides of the kettle, just before it reaches a rolling boil. Tea purists say that white tea is best infused when the water is at about 70°C and green and black teas around 85°C. For Oolong tea, on the other hand, hotter temperatures are critical to getting the top notes of flavour and fragrance, so use freshly boiled water.

A few of my favourite herbal teas

Wild rooibos (red bush) is a tea I didn't used to like, but I suspect it was because I'd only tried fusty bags from health food stores. I'm now a fan, as a good rooibos can be lovely. It doesn't belong to the tea family as it's a legume and is therefore 100 per cent caffeine free, which can be useful if caffeine isn't your thing or if you want to avoid stimulating effects.

Lemon verbena *(Aloysia triphylla)* (the French call it verveine) is a leafy herb with a wonderfully refreshing lemon flavour. Pop a good pinch in the pot and leave it to stand for three to five minutes. Traditionally lemon verbena is believed to help aid digestion and alleviate stress. Studies aren't conclusive, but I do find it calming when anxiety levels are going up.

Chamomile *(Matricaria recutita)* is a beautiful flower and makes a delicious infusion. Although you can buy chamomile in teabags, I find the tea they make bitter and fusty, far inferior to that made with the dried flowers. Chamomile has long been respected for its ability to soothe sore stomachs and is renowned as a gentle sleep aid.

English peppermint has the tradition of being a good digestive tea, and can be just the thing to sip after a meal, but if you have problems such as stomach ulcers you should watch that the tea isn't made too strong as mint can very occasionally aggravate symptoms. There is a world of difference between mint tea from small sources passionate about their product and the stale mint teabags available from the more usual outlets.

Steaming coffee

As with tea, I tend to be somewhat particular about the type of coffee I enjoy and when I drink it. Some people find that too much coffee can make them jittery and aggravate anxiety. Caffeine is a key component of coffee and the one we nutritionally tend to focus on, although energy drinks and tea contain some caffeine too. Even though studies are somewhat inconclusive and the physiological mechanisms behind the effects of caffeine can be a little complex, my philosophy is that if you're going to have a cup of coffee, make it a good one and cut out downing a coffee for the sake of it. This way you'll be able to enjoy coffee as part of your day, and glean a little caffeine hit which can be useful to get your body going in the morning or to help ease a headache or migraine ◆ . When you would usually have had that habitual, unnecessary, lousy-tasting coffee, you can replace it with water, which is by far the most hydrating and beneficial fluid. There is quite a lot of confusing information out there about caffeine sensitivity surrounding bones, heart disease and brain health, so I just want to highlight where the studies have got us to at the moment.

Read more on:
◆ *Pages 41–45*

Bones

While caffeine can have an impact on calcium absorption and bone metabolism, it seems that if we have a consistently good intake of calcium we can still enjoy a little caffeine. Therefore a coffee in our day isn't going to undo all the good work we're trying to achieve with our bones. However, I would say that the majority of people struggle to meet the recommended calcium intake, and if you have bad habits such as not exercising or smoking, you may need to increase the amount of calcium-rich foods you consume. If you're looking for one thing in your life you can do to help with your bones (especially if you've been told that you have low bone density), maybe keeping your coffee intake in check is one of them.

Heart health

When it comes to preventing heart disease, the relationship coffee has with our blood cholesterol levels and other heart disease risk factors is a little confusing, to say the least. Some studies show that in older people drinking coffee can actually offer protective effects against heart disease, while others show that heavy coffee drinkers may find that their risk of developing heart disease will be high. Some people with heart disease or other heart-related problems such as high blood pressure are told to cut out coffee altogether, as it can interfere with their medication. The long and short of it seems to be that if you have a couple of cups a day (the old mantra of moderation in everything springs to mind) then you're not putting your heart at any risk; however, watch what you're adding to the coffee. You could be introducing some saturated fat and calories if you're a cream or full-fat loving latte drinker, and sugar if you like it sweet.

Read more on: ◆ Page 149 ▲ Page 189

It has also been suggested that drinking decaffeinated coffee could lead to a rise in harmful cholesterol levels, which in turn can increase the risk of heart disease and diabetes ◆ . However there are hundreds of studies that do not show increased health risks associated with drinking caffeinated, and particularly decaffeinated, coffee. If you only drink one cup each day, these claims probably have little relevance because your daily coffee dose is relatively low.

Brain health

Studies have shown that being a coffee drinker could in fact help to preserve some of our cognitive function – probably due to its effect on the way chemicals transmit thoughts in our brain. Some studies even show that people who drink coffee have a decreased risk of developing Alzheimer's in later life ▲, but we need far more research to show consistent results before we start thinking that the coffee pot should be permanently by our sides. The other argument is that too much caffeine can adversely affect the way the brain works if you're struggling with mood disorders such as depression. As always, everyone is different, so if you love coffee have a couple a day, ideally in the morning, as although the evidence is mixed as to whether caffeine aggravates sleep disorders like insomnia, many people I treat do find that either only drinking coffee in the morning or stopping it altogether helps them sleep better.

Enjoying coffee at its best

If you're going to drink coffee, make it a good-quality one you will truly enjoy. I love espresso with a little milk (the French call it a noisette, while the Italians refer to it as a macchiato), but I also enjoy a slightly longer coffee made in either a filter or a cafetière. In the latter case if I'm at home I'll grind my own coffee beans. The trick with both filter and cafetière coffee is to drink it freshly made, ideally within the first 15 minutes as this gives you the best flavour. With filter coffee in particular, if you leave it standing on the hot plate it will turn bitter.

Taking it with milk is a personal choice – I prefer a touch of hot milk with an espresso and a little more with a filter or cafetière coffee, because it not only enables me to have a longer drink, but it also provides an opportunity to take in some calcium-rich milk. You can of course use soya or oat milk and other types of non-dairy milk, but they can often curdle if you put them into coffee when it's too hot.

Drinking water

Many research bodies advise us that we should be drinking six to eight glasses of fluid every day, which usually works out at about one to one and a half litres (4–6 cups), depending on how large the glasses are. I recommend that two and a half litres a day is the optimum amount of water we should be drinking, and I'm not alone – the World Health Organisation (WHO) recommends that women should drink over two litres (8½ cups) of water a day, with men needing closer to three litres (about 13 cups). You need even more if you live in a hot climate, have a very active job or work out a lot – a good guide to how much extra you need when you work out is to think about drinking roughly an extra litre per hour of hard exercise. Everyone is different in how much water they can comfortably drink, and when you push your water intake up you may spend a lot of time in the bathroom to begin with. Your body will get used to it, especially if you can stagger your water intake throughout the day – say a glass an hour.

Most nutritionists don't like to say whether we should be drinking water or other fluids such as juices, etc., but it's my experience that the more plain water you drink, the better your energy levels, your skin and digestive system will be; in fact the list of benefits is endless. It's fine to include the odd glass of fruit juice, tea or coffee but you can treat herbal teas in the same way as plain water. I would always say that the ideal amount of water should be drunk in the form of plain water or herbal teas, and anything else is extra. I realise that drinking two and a half litres (10 cups) of water and then putting tea and coffee on top of that is an awful lot, but it's something to aim for as I see so many people who feel great when they drink a similar amount (as I reach for yet another glass!).

It helps to have water on your desk when working, or a jug of water in a prominent place at home, as it serves as a constant reminder to drink. Try adding fresh mint, lemongrass or thin slices of cucumber, lemon, lime or orange to a jug of cold water, as these can infuse a subtle flavour and look pretty. It helps too to have a nice glass or mug instead of a plastic cup – all these little things make a difference to whether you're inclined to drink the water.

What kind of water?

If you totted up two and a half litres (10 cups) of water a day over a lifetime it would amount to a significant amount of money if you drank only bottled water. And the health benefits of bottled water versus tap water may surprise you – tap water is just as hydrating and healthy, so it's worth putting up with the odd snooty waiter's tut-tuts. The main water suppliers are under a legal obligation to maintain a safe drinking water supply to your house, so if you're concerned that the water that comes out of your tap doesn't taste right or isn't good for you, get in touch with your supplier. Bottled waters can have higher salt levels than many tap waters and don't offer the same fluoride protection. Water fluoridation is the addition of fluoride to our water supply to help prevent tooth decay. The World Health Organisation suggests a level of fluoride from 0.5 to 1.0mg per litre, depending on climate, but bottled water typically has unknown fluoride levels, and some domestic water filters remove some or all fluoride. But bottled waters can be more to your taste and can be more practical. And don't forget sparkling water, which I love to drink sometimes with meals.

If portability is a key concern, think about carrying around a flask or bottle filled with tap water. This is a much more environmentally friendly way to carry water around, without getting through large numbers of bottles, which need to be recycled or create waste. If the taste of the water that comes out of your tap isn't to your liking you could try a water filter (fitted to your tap or one of the smaller jug-style ones) or simply placing a jug of cold water in the fridge for a couple of hours can improve the flavour too. It's important to replace water filters as frequently as instructed by the manufacturer, to ensure that they continue to filter the water correctly and hygienically. If you have tap water or opened bottled water in the fridge, drink it within 24 hours, especially if you have been drinking it directly from the bottle. There are food poisoning bugs that like to hang around in stagnant water, which may be fine to shrug off when you're fit and healthy, but in the vulnerable, such as the young, old or unwell, could cause health problems. We consider water to be harmless and 99 per cent of the time it is, but we need to be careful, as with food, to store it correctly.

If you're looking for a non-dairy source of calcium, remember that if you live in a hard water area the calcium content of your tap water will be higher than in a soft water area. Bottled waters have to declare their calcium content, so look at their labels to see if there is a water higher in calcium that you like.

Being sensible about alcohol

Those wanting to drink sensibly should drink a maximum of two to three units a day (14 units a week) for women and three to four units a day (21 units a week) for men and avoid binge drinking. Drinking this amount of alcohol affords you all the benefits we often read about, such as reducing risk of heart disease, however it's a good idea to have one or two alcohol-free days during the week and to try to spread your weekly allowance out evenly. Despite several PR messages about beer containing antioxidants, red wine being the healthiest drink for your heart, and so on, let's just knock the implied notion of 'the more you drink the healthier you will be' on the head. There is no real evidence that red wine is better than any other alcohol, and resveratrol, the component concerned, may work well in a test tube but not so well in the body. Sorry to be the bearer of such news, but see it this way – choose the drink you enjoy and drink just a small amount for the pleasure and the health benefits, be this red wine, white wine or beer. Your body will react to alcohol in a unique and different ways, so watch how you drink it: it can disrupt sleep, lower energy and mood levels, and can for some be a strong contributory factor in carrying too much weight.

Alcohol is not only calorific but can also increase appetite, reduce your resolve to eat well and make you crave fatty and salty foods, which can easily be consumed in great quantities if you are in an alcohol haze. Eating salty crisps, nuts, olives, canapés or nibbles with alcoholic drinks makes us thirstier, as the body tries to get us to drink more water to enable it to get rid of the excess salt. We should quench this thirst with water and not another quaff of something alcoholic, as alcohol is also dehydrating. Food is good at helping to slow down the absorption of alcohol, but ideally, we should have something substantial and low in salt – the combination of salt and alcohol can make hangovers far worse.

I don't want to dwell on the negatives too much, but when we have stressful and busy lives it can be far too easy to slip into a habit of drinking too much alcohol. This is especially easy because many people still tend to assume that a glass of wine is just one unit, and it's not – it can be two or three units in the case of some of the enormous glasses that are used nowadays. Pints or half litres of beer can be easier to get a realistic check on how much you're drinking as they're a consistent measurement, but the alcohol content of beers and lagers can vary enormously and you need to bear this in mind when you decide what to drink.

Drinking alcohol on an empty stomach will make its effects more pronounced, as you need food to slow down its absorption into your body. Drinking plenty of water also reduces the effects of the alcohol, so maybe have a couple of glasses of water first and then enjoy wine or beer with your meal, with more water alongside. Be mindful that bubbles increase the speed of alcohol absorption, so champagne and sparkling wine often have the most dramatic alcoholic effects – and mixing drinks increases the chances of being hit with a hangover.

Alcohol and the mind

If you have problems controlling what you eat – whether it's wanting to binge on everything in the fridge or you are desperately trying to get a healthy eating routine going – my experience with treating patients is that alcohol can be a real menace. It can make you eat too much, as you seldom feel full at the right moment, and can dissipate all your good intentions. If you are prone to under-eating, alcohol can meddle with your thought processes and make you feel more anxious, colouring your perception of reality. So consider knocking alcohol on the head while you're trying to get a grip on food and the path of eating the right foods.

Headaches and migraines

At some time or other you're bound to get a headache, but sometimes they become frequent and you may suspect that they are more like migraines, which are typically experienced on one side of the head. Migraine sufferers experience visual auras, extreme pain, sickness and an inability to cope with bright lights and sounds. Physiologically headaches and migraines are very different and although we still don't really know what causes them, doctors believe that they are brought on by chemical changes in the brain's nerve cells. Many factors can trigger a migraine or headache, such as certain foods, tyramine, caffeine, MSG (a flavour enhancer found in many processed products and Chinese food), alcohol, hormonal changes in the menstrual cycle or stress. The first thing is to check with your doctor that the diagnosis is correct, and then it's a simple case of seeing what you can change in your lifestyle to reduce their frequency and ferocity.

The frustrating thing about headaches and migraines is that there are often so many contributing factors. Sometimes you can eat or drink a trigger food and be completely fine while at other times you'll be staying well away from them when a headache or migraine hits you. All we can do is identify and then eliminate as many of the triggers as possible – some being easier to deal with than others. Women in particular may find that they are more affected at particular times of the month, but keeping a food diary ◆ for a few weeks can help you to identify vulnerable times or general trends you can look at improving. This can equally apply to men, and can also be exacerbated when you have other lifestyle factors coming into play, such as greater pressures at work or home, or have to do a lot of travelling.

Read more on:
◆ *Page 11*

Roasted butternut squash & spicy sweetcorn soup, page 234

Tyramine

Tyramine is an amino acid that we naturally have in our body, but is also found in particular foods and drinks that may provoke headaches and migraines. Tyramine is mostly found in offal, mature cheese, peanuts, peanut butter, chocolate, broad beans, cured sausage, sauerkraut and herring (especially pickled). In fact as a broad stroke, anything fermented, pickled or marinated is best avoided.

Caffeine

The causes of headaches and migraines are ill understood and most people react in their own way to caffeine. What we do know is that caffeine in medication or drinking coffee with migraine medication can increase the speed at which the drug is absorbed, and therefore the rate at which your head starts to feel better.

What we also find is that if you dramatically cut down your caffeine intake you're likely to get a withdrawal headache, which sometimes triggers a migraine. I would suggest that if you are having a lot of caffeine-rich drinks and think they might be a contributing factor to your headaches or migraine, see if you can gradually cut them out rather than going cold turkey – try this over a few days and then, once you're down to two or three a day (a pretty good level to be at), you can enjoy a couple of espressos in the morning and a delicious cup of tea in the afternoon. This enables you to enjoy them, hopefully without exacerbating headaches, and if you keep at this level for a couple of weeks you will soon see if you feel any better. Some migraine or headache sufferers feel much better by not having anything caffeinated at all, while sometimes a cup of coffee or tea can prevent the first signs of a headache or migraine from getting worse.

Alcohol

We can be slightly more precise about alcohol. It's my experience not only from treating patients but also from being a migraine sufferer myself, that drinking alcohol on an empty stomach, or when dehydrated, exhausted or stressed, can also saddle you with an alarming headache or migraine. Although some people find that champagne and red wine are the worst offenders, for many others (myself included) white wine is worse. But it all depends on the type of grape and the additives, such as sulphites, which have been added. It's worth keeping a note of what you drink and how it affects you, as it could be a simple case of avoiding specific wines. Avoid mixing your drinks and line your stomach with food before, during and after drinking alcohol.

Unfortunately, alcoholic drinks don't have to declare their contents so you can't always find out what goes into them. (Note that it's worth keeping an eye on the labels of soft drinks too – even cordials such as elderflower – as they may contain sulphites.)

Keeping blood sugars within the comfort zone

It does seem that eating regularly and avoiding very sweet, high-GI (glycaemic index) foods can be a key contributing factor in managing or avoiding headaches and migraines. Some endocrinologists dismiss the notion that sugar can cause symptoms in people who don't have a hormonal problem such as diabetes, but this isn't what I see in myself or my patients. I find that the problem is exacerbated by eating very sweet or high-GI foods on an empty stomach. This means biscuits, cakes, sweets and sweet drinks ◆. If you absolutely crave a sweet snack, try pears, dried apricots, plums, grapes, dates or kiwi fruit, as these seem better tolerated, as does eating something sweet after a meal containing protein as the protein helps to slow down the absorption of the sugar, making its less pronounced.

Read more on:
◆ Pages 146–148

Skipping meals is a common trigger for headaches and migraines, especially breakfast. But this isn't an excuse for constant nibbling – three meals a day plus a couple of snacks should help you to get into a routine

Be mindful but not scared of salt

Official guidelines state that adults should eat less than 6g of salt a day (less for children). If you look at this amount on a teaspoon it is shockingly small and if you consider that most of us use a pinch when we're cooking, it can soon add up. Although I use a lot of alternative seasonings in my food – garlic, black pepper, fresh chilli, fresh herbs and spices, lemon juice – sometimes there are still moments when I reach for the salt and needn't feel guilty. But as a general rule, taste before you season and avoid putting salt on the table as this only adds to the temptation to grab some.

We need to strike a balance – the odd dip into some salted crisps, olives or smoked trout or salmon with capers isn't going to harm you, as the body easily steps into action and gets rid of the salt (in urine). I think that to vilify salt and reduce our intake so that food becomes bland can lead to overeating. If food is tasty and well seasoned it's usually easier to stop eating when you feel full. If food is boring it often takes more to hit the 'I'm satiated' bell. So in my mind, it's better to use it judicially, cutting it out gradually so that you learn to live with less.

I am not denying that there are worrying risks in having a diet that is high in salt. It has a profound impact on our heart, largely through aggravating blood pressure and if we reduce our salt intake by around 2.5g a day it could reduce the risk of stroke or heart attack by one quarter. But it's not just our hearts and brains that can suffer – high salt intake has been linked with osteoporosis and cancer, specifically of the stomach – so we do need to do something about it.

Having salty-tasting foods as treats only is an obvious way to go, but I suspect the real reason that salt is made such an issue in the health headlines is that in some sectors of the processed food industry there are far higher levels of salt than you would imagine (this is where Guideline Daily Amounts (% Daily Value) can be very useful on the labels of processed foods). Be careful if you find yourself heading towards the cheaper, economy lines, as some of them contain nasty surprises. Some supermarkets are able to sell them for less because they fill sausages, meat pies, ready-meals and ready-made sandwiches with cheaper filler ingredients such as flour, starch, etc., but since these are pretty bland in their own right, some manufacturers whack in hefty amounts of salt to make them appetising.

One of the most shocking examples is breakfast cereals. They're traditionally seen as sweet foods, but the high sugar content fools the taste buds into not clocking the fact that there can be a lot of salt in them too. Porridge and natural wholegrains generally have low levels of salt, but there are a lot of others that don't, so be particularly vigilant with processed foods – the labels will help.

Among other things, too much salt can aggravate high blood pressure, bone loss and fluid retention. Because our taste buds can fade in their accuracy, we may think we need more salt to make food appetising, which is a problem. Not only will we eat more processed foods, which will often contain a lot of salt, but if we're shaking the salt cellar over food that has been salted beforehand, we are probably taking in too much.

of preventing headaches. If you feel a migraine coming on, try to have something bland, for example a couple of rice cakes or a slice of toast and a glass or two of water, as sometimes this can lessen the severity. If nausea is a problem, just try a few mouthfuls and then rest to let the food settle – sometimes a very small amount of food can really help. Relaxing is beneficial too – but this is not to say that exercising won't be a good thing in your life, as it can be a good stress-reliever. As with most things, having regular sleeping times – both going to sleep and waking – can help as a lifestyle measure.

Cellulite

Contrary to popular thinking, physiologically, cellulite isn't any different to any other sort of fat and therefore isn't caused by toxins per se – it's just one of those very annoying aspects of being a woman. However, it isn't just a female issue and can be the bane of men's lives too – some adults will spend a fortune on creams, potions, brushes and massages to try to reduce the orange peel-like skin around their thighs. When it comes to food and drink, you should find that eating a nourishing diet, light in calories and high in fruits and vegetables, should pay off. It's also especially helpful if you can incorporate fat burning exercises. As much as I'd love to conjure up a miracle here, there aren't any specific cellulite-banishing foods, despite the claims made for foods such as grapefruit.

Depression

There is growing evidence to show that if we eat a well balanced and nourishing diet we are less likely to develop depression. Scientists believe in some cases it could be conected to an over-heated immune system – recasting depression as an inflammatory condition like heart disease or rheumatoid arthritis. But the symptoms of depression are very varied, as is the degree to which we suffer, and so while not eating well can be a contributing factor, it would be wrong to imply that all depression is caused simply by what we do or don't eat.

Depression is clinically defined in many textbooks and I don't want to dwell on the medical aspects of this illness, but from a nutritional perspective over the years I have often (but not always) seen that by changing the foods we eat we can influence our moods and reduce the other classic symptoms, such as poor sleep, low energy and disturbed appetite. Appetite can go either way – putting us off all foods or eating compulsively to try to make ourselves feel better. Depression can make us crave different foods, which can knock out supplies of other nutrients in the body.

A lot of anti-depressant medication can disrupt the way we eat. Some suppress appetite and if our excess weight is an exacerbating factor in feeling low about ourselves, losing a few pounds and getting in control of what we eat can be a huge factor in helping us to work our way out of a depression. Other anti-depressants can make us crave foods, which if we've been on the underweight end of the weight spectrum can be a useful tool to make us eat something, particularly if we have been suffering from an eating disorder ◆. But more commonly, some anti-depressant medication can both make us crave overly sweet foods and all the starchy stuff to such a great extent that weight gain becomes a problem. This can be a real hurdle for some people, especially women, who I've found can be reluctant to take anti-depressant medication if it's going to make them put on weight.

Read more on:
◆ Pages 160–161
▲ Pages 66–67
● Pages 170–171

Easy apple & greengage strudel, page 247

But nine times out of ten, if we can improve the balance of nutrients in our diet, the symptoms improve and in some cases we may be able to stop or reduce taking the medication. In any case check whether you're meant to take drugs on an empty stomach or with meals and discuss with your doctor if your medication is adversely affecting your appetite. Do keep in contact with your doctor or therapist, as it's good to keep them in the loop and to let them know if your weight is changing, as your dose of medication may need to be adjusted. I mention this because sometimes we think that doctors won't be interested in what we eat, but in fact by keeping them informed you can ensure that your medical care is appropriate and working.

It's also important to establish from your doctor's assessment whether there are nutrition-related factors which may well be causing you to feel low, such as iron deficiency anaemia ▲ or coeliac disease ●. Certain drugs taken for other health problems, such as some blood pressure medication and particular contraceptive pills, can have mood-lowering effects too, and your doctor can ensure that you're receiving the right help.

If you just don't feel like eating

Although in times of plenty our bodies lay down stores of many nutrients, which we can draw on when we're not eating so well, if the days of not eating much or well turn into weeks and months, over time our nutrient stores can become depleted. As I've mentioned before, a lack of iron can

Read
more on:
◆ Page 19

Pearled spelt
with broad
beans,
asparagus
& dill,
page 208

lead to iron deficiency anaemia, which in itself can cause many of the classic depressive symptoms such as lethargy, low mood and disrupted sleep. Lack of the B vitamins ◆ too can cause depression, as can not eating enough selenium, a mineral that we most commonly find in fruits and vegetables.

The long and the short of it is that if we're off our food and are not eating a diet rich in all the vitamins, minerals and other nutrients our body needs, we can soon start to feel low. Rather frustratingly, appetite can go, which is in fact the opposite of what we really need our bodies to feel – it would be handy if our natural survival instincts kicked in and we started craving the foods that would nourish us and replenish the stores, but often this just doesn't happen. The less we eat the less we feel like eating – and this is particularly common in people who don't have appetising food available to them. Out of sight, out of mind, is a real problem for people who live on their own or are the ones who have traditionally been the cooks. Having to cook for someone else can help, as it stops us slumping into the 'I won't bother putting anything together' phase. So often if you can just get past the first mouthful, your appetite will kick in and you may find you actually enjoy eating.

It helps to stick to three meals a day with a couple of snacks in between, as one of the mistakes that some people with depression make is just snacking on biscuits and other easy-to-grab foods, which takes away the appetite for a proper meal. If you just feel like eating bowls of pasta and mashed potatoes, or having slice after slice of toast, this is fine in the short term – a few days of eating like this isn't going to harm you, and indeed it's much better to be eating something rather than nothing. But in the medium to long term, your body and your brain in particular won't benefit as much. So if you can, try to find something you feel like eating, even if it's putting tomatoes and cucumber into a sandwich or throwing tinned sweetcorn and frozen spinach into an omelette – this way you'll start to build up the spectrum of nutrients we know help your body to perform at its best.

As to how you manage the practical aspects of shopping and cooking, it will depend largely on what works. Sometimes it can help to try the main weekly shop option, so that you stock up on foods and can then simply throw something easy together with little effort. This can work especially well if you're more of a planner – writing out a week's meal plan can help some people shop well and persuade them into eating food they perhaps wouldn't have thought about on the shopping day.

On the other hand, buying food on an almost daily basis can help to cut down on food wastage and, depending on the shops you choose, be just what you need to get your appetite going; for example, seeing the food – a fresh pasta sauce in a deli, for instance – or asking the advice of a passionate procurer or food shop owner, can give you an idea of what's good and how you could cook it. I'd try both ways of organising your shopping and eating, and perhaps also look online for a few inspiring small suppliers who could send you something delicious ◆.

Read more on:◆ Pages 21–25

Sometimes it helps to invite a close friend to eat with you, as the added dimension of having to put something together for them can make you feel more inclined to be creative and eat something better than a slice of toast. You could also ask or take up the offer of a friend who's a good cook to bring something round or to stock up your freezer with a few nourishing dishes. It doesn't have to be anything complicated – a few batches of bolognese sauce or ratatouille can be great for times when you just can't muster the enthusiasm to make anything for yourself. Don't forget that many people love being asked to do something practical, and can feel chuffed that you like their cooking enough to ask them – so often those around us feel useless when someone they care about is suffering from depression, and if you can give them the task of cooking something nutritious then this is a win-win situation. If you have the inclination to cook yourself, make more than you can eat in one meal and put some in the freezer or fridge ▲.

If you find your weight spiralling out of control

The first thing to do is to check with your doctor to see if weight gain is a side-effect of any medication you're taking. If it's impossible to change drugs, the likelihood is that the physiological, metabolic changes that have led to your weight gain will have a ceiling in their effect – it's often only at the beginning of taking a new drug. Of course there are instances when you may have been through a particularly anxious or severe depressive spell and you've been eating well but have still lost weight. If the drug you're taking or the therapy that you're receiving enables you to feel happier and less anxious the simple fact that you're feeling better means your body won't be continually burning up food and will start to feel that it can relax. So if you continue to eat the same amount of food your weight will slowly start to creep back on.

I wouldn't recommend for anyone, but particularly when you're suffering from depression, the idea of trying to eat what's commonly referred to in the media as a cleanse or detox or a very low-calorie diet, as your body needs good nourishment when you're depressed, and depriving yourself can leave you feeling depleted in every sense. It can also change the way your body metabolises medication, which could unsettle your regime. This is not to say that things like cutting out the very sweet and fatty stuff and, say, drinking more water and fewer artificial drinks shouldn't be attempted, as I've often seen that patients who take control of what they eat and have a nourishing, healthy diet can get themselves out of a depressive dip. Of course taking charge of your eating also gives you a practical strategy, something you can build into your day-to-day plan, which can be a really positive way to help get you through depression.

Read more on:
◆ Page 11
▲ Pages 40–41

Chicken with winter vegetables, page 214

It can help to keep a food diary ◆ for a few weeks, to monitor simple things like ensuring that you're eating regularly and drinking enough water as these can be things we lose track of. Alcohol is a depressant as well as an appetite stimulant (and can also be contraindicated with some anti-depressant medication), so see if you can cut down on the amount you drink. Alcohol can also exacerbate many of the symptoms of depression and can cause you to feel out of control if eating disorders or bingeing are a current issue or if you've struggled with them in the past – it can play havoc with your perception of what you have or haven't eaten, and staying away from it can be one big thing that could help ▲.

I hate it when doctors pooh-pooh the notion that changing eating habits is a useless thing to try for people suffering with depression, as my experience shows quite the opposite. In an illness where so much structure can be lost, and the depression can take such an overwhelming hold on day-to-day life, it's helpful to be able to focus on something which is not only practical for the individual but, as I mentioned before, for those around them to be able to feel they're doing something useful. If you can provide the body with good, nourishing meals all sorts of depression-related symptoms can disappear or at least lessen in their severity. In my opinion it's incredibly important for anyone who's suffering from any level of depression to be given the right nutritional support – if you look at the cost of so many aspects of managing depression and other types of mental illness, the costs of eating the right food pale into insignificance, and let's not forget that so much can be communicated and gained on an emotional level from eating delicious nourishing foods. As John Gunther said, 'All happiness depends on a leisurely breakfast', which is reiterated in the Jewish proverb that states, 'Worries go down better with soup.'

Nurturing a New Life

Making the decision to have a child is a momentous one for many women. As Elizabeth Stone once said, 'It is to decide forever to have your heart go walking around outside your body.' Becoming pregnant or deciding to be a mum to a child is an enormous and gorgeous, if overwhelming, concept. It's a time when our body changes, along with our moods, our relationships and how we see the world.

The changes to our body in pregnancy, and the responsibility we have for providing the right nourishment for a new life, can be somewhat daunting. We can begin to feel the need to start looking at food under a microscope, and see meal planning as a military exercise. This is a shame, as other than the foods we need to avoid (because they carry a high risk of food-poisoning bacteria, which in the case of listeria and salmonella can cause untold damage to an unborn child), we simply need to eat nutritious food with just a few tweaks to meet the additional demands of a growing baby. So the aim of this chapter is to take you through what is best to eat to keep you both as strong and healthy as possible, to support a plentiful nourishing supply of breast milk and to get your body back in to shape.

Trying to get pregnant

Getting pregnant can be the easiest thing in the world for some couples while for others it seems an impossibly difficult and upsetting hurdle to overcome. While fertility treatments such as IVF are miracle-makers when all other efforts have failed, there are many cases where looking at lifestyle can be the first stop to help a couple with conception. The strong relationship that exists between exercise, drinking, eating, and how you cope with stress and juggle the demands of everyday life is so powerful that more often than not fertility specialists will recommend that you look into them before you head down the route of assisted fertility treatment. Even if you are already receiving an additional drug or procedure, you should pay attention to how you live, as all the areas covered in this chapter have a role to play. And of course the guidelines apply to every couple trying for a family, whether with treatment or without.

There are definite relationships between conceiving a healthy baby and parents who have enough of the specific nutrients that I discuss throughout this chapter. It's important, however, to keep the role that food plays in perspective as there are many different aspects involved in conceiving a child. If you get all het up and start treating your eating and drinking habits as a military operation, it is only going to make you both pretty miserable, which is hardly conducive to getting pregnant. It's a fine and often difficult line to tread between eating and living well to maximise your chances of conceiving, and allowing yourself a relaxed and fun Friday night.

When you're planning and trying to conceive, a good starting point is to look at the real way you eat and drink, not just what you think you do, as there can be a big difference between the two – we all fool ourselves at times! Keep a food diary for a couple of weeks ◆. I know it's cumbersome, but I guess you've probably started thinking about your life in weeks if not days: is it a good day to have sex or not? So a food diary in which you record not just what you eat but also how much shouldn't be too arduous a task. Then you can see what you're doing and work through a few points where you can improve the chances of getting pregnant. And looking at your diet isn't just worth doing if you're a woman – men need to take note, as eating well can improve the quality and quantity of sperm produced, as well as food and drink having an impact on libido for you both. I see many couples in my practice who are desperate to conceive and want to explore how nutritional supplements can improve their chances, but studies show time and time again that your body is best nourished from eating a well-balanced diet.

Read more on: ◆ Page 11

Non-food changes that increase the chances of conceiving

- **Stop smoking:** Smoking has been linked to both infertility and early menopause in women and to sperm problems in men. It also reduces the success of fertility treatments.
- **Be active:** Keeping active, with at least 30 minutes of cardiovascular moderate-intensity exercise a day (working out at the gym, swimming, cycling, or brisk walking), helps you stay fit and produces endorphins that boost mood. Many patients of mine also find that when they start exercising on a regular basis they feel more positive about their bodies, so that libido increases – there's nothing like feeling more toned and less wobbly for getting you in the mood! Weight is far easier to keep under control with some calorie expenditure. Watch, though, that the exercise doesn't become too intensive and obsessive, as too much can exhaust a pressurised and stressed body and low body fat levels can upset the reproductive hormone cycles.
- **Keep cool:** For men it's particularly important to keep cool – for optimum sperm production the testicles need to be a couple of degrees cooler than the rest of the body. So it's best to avoid tight underwear and jeans, saunas and steaming hot baths.
- **Relax:** Try to reduce stress levels as much as possible. Although stress doesn't cause infertility, being overly worried and stressed can adversely affect menstrual cycles and also lower libido. So try to build in some 'you' time that's relaxed – try not to get overly anxious and controlling over eating and living the right lifestyle, as this is counterproductive.
- **Avoid drugs:** Recreational drugs such as marijuana and cocaine affect sperm counts, as do some prescription drugs – both men and women can have their chances of conception reduced by certain drugs, so discuss this with your doctor if you're taking regular medication. Being exposed to certain paints or pesticides within an industrial workplace may also affect sperm quality.

Body weight and fertility

Read
more on:
◆ Page 116

Broad bean
& pistachio
hummus,
page 227

The consensus of opinion is that being over or underweight can disrupt your periods and hinder conception, which is why we encourage anyone trying to get pregnant to have a body mass index (BMI) of between 20 and 25 ◆. However, it's more subtle than just what women weigh, as fertility can also be affected by the amount of fat that's carried (as in percentage). This means that even if you're of ideal weight it can be worth looking at your diet and the way you exercise to see if you can reduce your body fat content to within the range of 20–25 (the average body fat content of women is about 28 per cent). You may be surprised when you step on either a scale, which is able to measure the percentage body fat, or get the trainer in your local gym to do some simple measurements to give you an indication of whether they think your body fat level is too high. The likelihood is that if you have a BMI within the ideal range your fat percentage won't be far out, but it's worth looking to see if you can change the way the fat is distributed by exercising well.

But at the other end of the weight and body fat spectrum, being underweight has a profound effect on fertility – your body is at its most fertile when it has a body fat content of around 22 per cent, as the fat is needed to support the manufacture of the necessary hormones to enable you to ovulate and menstruate. If you have a BMI of less than 19, it's worth checking your body fat percentage to see whether you need to increase the amount and variety of the foods you eat. Your body fat percentage isn't usually lower than this unless you're either on the very skinny side, or are suffering from a condition, an eating disorder like anorexia, or a phobia of eating well. But it's also possible to have too low a level of body fat if you're a sports fanatic, and although you have a normal BMI the fact is that you're made up of too much muscle and not enough fat.

Mother nature needs you to have enough fat prior to conception to be able to support a healthy pregnancy, and afterwards – if you decide – to enable you to breastfeed since the milk is largely produced from your fat stores. The desire to be a mum can sometimes be just what you need to get you out of the routine of not eating enough or over-exercising. If you're underweight prior to or while you're pregnant you also have a higher chance of giving birth to a baby with too low a body weight and all the health problems this can bring into play, such as higher rates of heart disease and type 2 diabetes in later life. I don't mean to scare you by this, just give you some extra encouragement should you need it: if you can get your body weight and body fat levels up to a good level to support you both during pregnancy, not only are you going to be giving your baby the best possible start in life but you will also be strong enough once you've given birth to enjoy being a mum.

A word of reassurance, too, that while there are some women who blame being overweight on having children, which can scare the living daylights out of anyone who thinks that being an overweight mum is the last thing you want be, be comforted by the fact that there is no reason why you can't return to having a great body after giving birth if you eat and exercise well. It's the change in eating habits and motivational issues that influence how successful a woman is at getting her body back into shape; the only physiological issue that has any impact great enough to be important is breastfeeding – you can generally lose weight more successfully. So if you're worried that getting pregnant means you will turn into a hippopotamus and not be able to get your body back, this isn't going to happen unless you eat too much during pregnancy and don't do any exercise.

The dad-to-be's diet

Read more on:
♦ Pages 18–21

My mum's chicken pie, page 211

Generally, the dad-to-be's diet should be every bit as balanced, varied and nutritious as that of the mum-to-be. As a future dad it helps to ensure your diet includes zinc, folates and other foods rich in antioxidants, such as vitamin C ♦. All of these help your body to make normal functioning sperm. Great sources of zinc include dark chicken meat and lean red meat, shellfish, milk and dairy foods, bread, baked beans and good cereal products – so if you need an excuse to enjoy a good-quality lean steak this is it! It's tempting to think that supplements could further increase your zinc intake and therefore your chances of conceiving, but studies don't show this – however, if you're not much of a meat lover you could take a supplement containing 15mg of zinc each day.

Vitamin C is best gleaned from a diet rich in fresh fruit and vegetables. Not only does your body absorb vitamin C from fruits and vegetables (frozen vegetables and fruits can be a very practical and rich source of vitamin C too), but the nutrient package within these foods provides other useful fertility-associated nutrients such as folate. People are often astounded by how little vitamin C we actually need in our diet to meet our body's requirement – it's only 60mg a day, which you can easily hit by eating an orange or a small (125ml/4oz) glass of orange juice. So as you can see, if you're managing to eat the recommended five portions of fruit and veg in a day – say having a bowl of fresh fruit in the morning and then salads and vegetables as a significant part of your two other meals – it's easy to meet your body's vitamin requirements without a pill in sight. Smoking reduces your body's ability to absorb vitamin C, so try to knock it on the head.

Fertility treatment

Infertility is thought to affect about one in seven couples – most of the women will eventually become pregnant naturally, but waiting can be frustrating and upsetting, while a significant minority will not be successful after years of trying. Often the treatment of infertility involves taking drugs, which can have side effects in varying degrees depending on the treatment you receive and your body's ability to cope – some women find them more upsetting than others and it's impossible to tell how your body will react. The most common reported side-effects for taking drugs orally include abdominal bloating, nausea, breast tenderness, hot flushes and mood changes. At a time when you could really do with feeling at your best, since IVF and other fertility treatments are invasive and stressful enough, the drugs themselves can play havoc with your body. However, these effects can often be improved and managed by looking at the way you eat and drink.

I'm not going to say that food can be a miracle cure, but many women I've treated do seem to find that tweaking the way they eat can take the sting out of the treatment and help them to feel more 'normal' and like the person they want to be. For instance, if you're feeling bloated, it could just be that something as simple as cutting down on the amount of wheat-based foods you eat and including more rice, beans and lentils could help. After all, a large tummy is the last thing you want if there are people around you who know you're trying to get pregnant before you've been successful.

If you're feeling sick a lot, watch that you don't fall into the trap of not eating much. Eat small nourishing meals, maybe juggling the time of day when you have your main meal – often it can suit you better to have this at lunchtime instead of in the evening. If you find that breakfast is a no-no, as you're just feeling too sick to eat anything, don't stress about it. You can make up for it during the rest of the day – maybe have a brunch which is more substantial. Some women also feel that for their body to change and make them feel lousy is unfair, especially when many of the drug side-effects are similar to actually being pregnant. Even if you're trying to relax and not think about getting pregnant every minute of every day, your body may be continually reminding you that you're not. It's a lot to deal with, so if making changes to what and how you eat makes you feel better, it can be a positive and empowering thing to take control of. If you find yourself craving sweet food, try to restrict the high-GI ◆ options as they seldom make you feel great bar the initial buzz – it's much better to choose something nourishingly sweet. Some women find that sniffing a vanilla pod can take away their sweet cravings – strange but it can work!

Read more on:
◆ Pages 146–148

Pearled spelt with broad beans, asparagus & dill, page 208

Inspiring vegetables

- Samphire can be bought from fish stalls in markets or from good online grocers. Simply steam it and then marinate in a herby dressing. It's delicious with fish and roasted meats, or a few slices of charcuterie and warm bread.
- Golden and yellow beetroot are wonderful in salads, especially when roasted. Mashed beetroot on toast is delicious too, topped with sliced tomatoes and a dollop of hummus.
- When you're making a salad dressing mix the ingredients over a gentle heat and pour over the salad leaves while still warm. You can either eat it straight away, in which case you will benefit from the aromas of the warmed oil, or alternatively if it's a salad made from vegetables such as beans or roasted vegetables let the vegetables marinate in the dressing for a few hours and then eat them at room temperature. If you like a hint of sweetness in your salad dressing, try using maple syrup. It has a far more complex flavour than sugar, so the dressings have an interesting note.
- Experiment with tapenades and herb and spice blends such as harissa. You can use them to roast vegetables, in which case they can be rubbed in or stirred through like a marinade.
- If you're making a salad as a main meal and fancy a cheese hit but don't want to use much, finely crumble a cheese such as feta or a Wensleydale or Lancashire cheese into it. Alternatively, grate a good Pecorino or Parmesan cheese very finely.
- Be more courageous with chillies – there are so many different varieties with varying strengths of kick. Just a quarter of a teaspoon of freshly chopped chilli can impart a warming kick to a salad dressing, marinade or stir-fry. Using flavours such as chilli or freshly ground pink peppercorns instead of black means that you find yourself using less salt. The more complex flavours you use, the more your taste buds will be stimulated and the more satisfied you'll be after your meal.
- Traditionally, western cuisine has not been the most adventurous in using fresh herbs, and when we do use them we tend to use just one – mint with lamb, sage with pork, tarragon with chicken, etc. Try mixing a few together, as you can get some very good combinations. I particularly like mixing fresh basil, dill and parsley in a salad. Mint goes well with basil too – a tip here is to use a plastic knife or tear the leaves, as metal knives turn them black.
- Add fruit to salads, for example wafer-thin segments of very fresh orange, apple, pear, fig, peach, plum, or something more exotic such as pomegranate. Vegetables which are technically fruits, such as peppers, go well in salads, particularly if they're roasted.

Eating well in pregnancy

The old wives' tale of eating for two has long been discredited, as although our body needs some extra calories each day (and a few extra milligrams of some essential vitamins like folic acid, and minerals such as iron and calcium), there's only one place that eating enough for two will take us – being fed up and looking and feeling like a beached whale. The physiological reality is that, although we need extra calories as our pregnancy progresses, we will become less active as we can't dart around in the same way, so our body just doesn't burn up as many calories. However, it should also be said that many of my pregnant patients do confess to at long last being able to step out of the food jail they've been in – a place of always feeling they should be slim. Finally, they can eat and not feel guilty. And why not? As long as you don't overdo it, enjoy this time of your life.

Pregnancy can be the perfect time to instil some good, nutritious eating habits if you've previously relied on your body's good will to put up with fast living, too much drinking, and bad eating. You may need to wait until after the first trimester, if nausea ◆ is preventing you from being able to stomach anything more than white toast (which, by the way, can be a very nourishing food to eat, try not to worry too much that you're not managing to get through your five-a-day, etc., as the amazing thing about pregnancy is that your baby will take what it needs from your stores. Also, your pregnant body will soon cotton on to the fact that it needs to be extra efficient at absorbing the essential nutrients from smaller amounts of food. The one person who loses out if this continues is you, the mum, as it can leave you deficient in minerals such as iron. Iron deficiency anaemia ▲ is particularly risky during the last trimester of your pregnancy, when the baby draws on your iron stores to support its rapid growth spurts.

If you've not managed to eat well during pregnancy, you can end up feeling depleted after the birth when your body really needs to be feeling strong; be this to support breastfeeding (which we know to be the best possible start for your baby), or to keep up with the constant demands of being a new mum.

Essentially when you're pregnant you should try to eat in the same way as you would normally – a good balance and spectrum of all the foods featured in the eat well plate ●. The calories you require to support your baby's growth and development aren't the same throughout the whole of the pregnancy – most of the extra is needed during the second and third trimesters. Try to hold back and just eat as normal

Read
more on:
◆ Pages
67–69
▲ Pages
66–67
● Page 14

during the early months, and this will help stave off feeling too enormous later on.

Studies show you only need an extra 200kcals per day during the third trimester, and if you bear in mind that this more or less equates to a sandwich made from a couple of thin slices of wholemeal bread with something like lean ham inside, or a large banana and an apple, you'll see that it isn't very much. If you've been struggling with gaining enough weight, say if you're suffering with sickness, have always been on the light side or continue to lead a very active life, you may need slightly more than this. Really the best way to check whether you're eating the right amount is to keep an eye on your weight – a gain throughout the three trimesters of about 12kg (26½ lb) is about right. Of course, there are lots of individual variations in weight gain and 12kg is an average. If you're heavier to start with you may gain less, whereas if your pre-pregnancy weight was on the low side, you may gain more. Some weeks your weight won't change much, but keep in touch with your obstetrician and health team so that they can help monitor your baby's growth and development and see how you're thriving too. If you find you are gaining more than is desirable, try to reduce the frequency of your snacks, take time to sit and savour your food, make sure you're not trying to quench thirst with food, keep a food diary ◆, try eating and exercising at different times and watch that you're not eating too many high-fat, high-sugar foods.

Read more on:
◆ Page 11
Beans with tomato, coriander & coconut milk, page 206

Safe eating in pregnancy

One of the most important things to watch out for when you're pregnant is that the foods you eat are safe for the two of you. This means looking at how you choose, prepare and cook produce in order to reduce the risk of exposing your unborn baby to both food-poisoning organisms (such as salmonella and listeria) and toxic food components. You also need to pay attention to the alcohol and caffeine you drink, and also at which nutritional supplements you take, as some just aren't suitable when you're expecting.

This can all sound alarming, but once you've read the fine print of the few things to avoid and how to reduce the risk it's pretty simple. It has astounded me over the years that some pregnant women who have fought tooth and nail to get pregnant ask me which foods to avoid only to then try to persuade me into saying it's okay for them to eat something they shouldn't. They just don't realise that during pregnancy, the bacterial infection that can arise from eating a food which contains listeria, for example, is extremely serious and life-threatening for the baby – it's not just a question of being off-colour for a couple of days. Yes, it's a shame not to have a soft-boiled egg and soldiers, but peace of mind is worth far more.

What a mum eats whilst pregnant (and breastfeeding) is also a factor in whether their child suffers from eczema. Although the studies show mixed results, there is some evidence to suggest that if you eat a diet rich in fruits and vegetables, especially those rich in beta carotene (the orange red and yellow fruits and vegetables) you are less likely to give birth to a child with eczema. Interestingly another recent study showed that if you have a diet rich in vitamin E such as olive oil and avocados ◆ your baby is less likely to suffer from an allergy-type wheeze. Rather than thinking you need to start measuring levels of these specific nutrients, I'd just treat research like this as encouragement to nourish your body as well as you can throughout pregnancy. If you have a particular worry over eczema (perhaps if you have a strong history of atopic eczema and allergies in your family), then it could be worth you taking an omega-3 supplement containing 2g (2,000 mg) combination of EPA and DHA, which has also been shown to be protective against developing eczema in the first year of life if taken whilst pregnant.

Read more on:
◆ *Pages 18, 101 & 104*

Listeria

Listeriosis can cause miscarriage, stillbirth, birth defects or severe illness once your baby is born. Foods to avoid are pâté, mould-ripened soft cheese, such as Brie and Camembert, blue-veined cheeses such as Stilton, unpasteurised milk and milk products. Hard cheeses such as Cheddar or other cheeses made from pasteurised milk, such as mozzarella, cottage cheese and processed cheese spreads, are all fine. Hard goat's cheeses are also fine to eat – it's the soft, chèvre-like ones you need to avoid. If you fancy your cheese soft, melt it on toast.

Listeria bacteria are destroyed by heat, and you should always, but particularly when you're pregnant, thoroughly heat food as per the instructions. Don't reheat ready-prepared meals, especially if they contain poultry. The real bane, I think, is having to avoid ready-prepared salads and cold dishes which you won't be reheating before you eat – quiches, flans and cold meat pies. If you buy salad leaves, wash them thoroughly in lots of running cold water and do the same with all fruits and vegetables in order to reduce the risk of contracting listeria.

Salmonella

Salmonella is the most common cause of food-poisoning and in severe cases can cause miscarriage or premature labour. Salmonella poisoning is most likely to come from raw eggs or uncooked poultry, so you need to stick to hard-boiled eggs avoiding raw or partially cooked eggs and all products containing them such as homemade mayonnaise, soufflés and custards. However, you can eat commercially produced mayo, as these almost always use pasteurised egg and don't contain any raw egg ingredients – but check the labels to make sure. It's possible to buy certain classifications of eggs from hens that have been vaccinated against salmonella, but this doesn't mean they are salmonella-free, so you still need to avoid eating them raw etc.

With poultry in particular you need to make sure that it's cooked all the way through – slicing through a chicken breast to check there are no cool spots. A chicken brick is one of the best ways to ensure that the chicken is well cooked but not dried out and rubbery. You need to watch how you handle raw poultry too – washing your hands thoroughly afterwards. And pay attention to how you store raw and cooked foods in your fridge, so that you don't get any cross-contamination from dripping raw chicken ◆ .

Read more on:
◆ *Pages 21–23*

Toxoplasmosis

Toxoplasmosis is caused by the organism Toxoplasma gondii, which can be found in raw meat, unpasteurised milk and cat faeces. If you contract it when you're pregnant it can, in rare cases, infect your baby via the placenta and lead to severe abnormalities such as blindness and brain damage. To reduce the risk of contracting it you need to avoid eating all raw and undercooked meat – steaks should be well cooked all the way through. Cooking it should be fine, but you need to be extra vigilant in washing your hands and wiping down surfaces. You also need to steer clear of unpasteurised milk and milk products (this is particularly the case with goat's milk). Give the job of cleaning out the cat litter tray to someone else or wear gloves if you have to do it. The same applies if you're gardening – always cover your hands so that they're not coming into contact with the soil. Ideally (although this is often impractical) the cat should go elsewhere for the few months of your pregnancy or be kept out of the kitchen, as they can transmit bacteria just by walking on kitchen surfaces.

Campylobacter

Campylobacter is one of the most common forms of food-poisoning, but if you contract it while pregnant it can cause miscarriage, stillbirth and induce premature labour. The most common sources of infection are poultry, unpasteurised milk and milk products, domestic pets and soil, so if you take the precautions listed above, you will reduce your risk. But you should also be careful with untreated water – both drinking it and coming into direct contact with it – and soil. Gardening gloves need to be on the shopping list from day one.

Peanuts

Twenty years ago peanuts weren't an issue, but it appears that peanut allergy is increasing in both adults and children. An allergic reaction can cause anaphylaxis, which is extremely serious and requires emergency treatment because the symptoms of respiratory obstruction and shock develop so quickly. We don't really know why this happens: some say we're bringing up our children in too clean and sterile an environment, which means that their immune systems don't develop the right level of response; others blame the use of more and more peanuts and peanut oil in our diet – Asian cuisine, which uses peanuts in many of its dishes, is playing a more prominent place in our eclectic tastes for food. Peanut oil is also being used in food and skin preparations, all of which concerns some immunologists enough to wonder if this is to blame.

It can all seem confusing, and we don't have the answers yet, but what we do know is that unless you have a strong history of allergies, such as asthma or eczema, in either of the parents' families, you should continue to eat peanuts while pregnant and breastfeeding as there is no evidence that this will cause your child to develop a peanut allergy. Even if you do have a family history of peanut allergy, there is no clear evidence to say if eating or not eating peanuts during pregnancy will affect the chance of your baby developing a peanut allergy. And in fact there is some evidence to suggest that by not including small amounts of peanuts in your diet, your unborn baby is unable to develop a tolerance to nut proteins, and you could be increasing the risk of the allergy developing. If you look at cultures where nuts are endemic within their cuisine from an early age, you seldom find peanut allergies.

Vitamin A

Although vitamins are vital for our overall health when it comes to being pregnant, you need to watch the amount of vitamin A you consume as high levels can be toxic and cause problems for your baby's growth and development. You not only need to steer well clear of any nutritional supplements containing vitamin A (such as cod liver oil), unless specifically prescribed by your doctor, but you also need to avoid foods that are naturally rich in this vitamin, namely liver and liver products such as pâté and liver sausage. Normal sausages are fine, as they're not full of liver – the liver is where the vitamin A is stored in animals and is therefore potentially toxic to unborn babies.

Drinking the right fluids

Read more on:
◆ Page 68

As well as watching your alcohol intake ◆ , it's wise to check that you're not drinking too much tea, coffee and other drinks such as cola, as all of these hit high on the caffeine stakes. Although the evidence isn't conclusive, too much caffeine for women may well lower the chance of conceiving. Caffeine intake during pregnancy should be limited to 200mg a day, which works out roughly (although amounts vary between types of coffee, etc.) at three mugs of instant coffee, six cups of tea or eight cans of cola a day. I know it sounds a lot, but if you had a couple of mugs of coffee, a can of coke and a chocolate bar in one day you'd already be almost up to the limit.

One theory suggests that stimulants affect ovulation by causing changes in hormone levels, which in turn hampers conception. In contrast, caffeine may actually help men's fertility by stimulating sperm motility; although the evidence again isn't conclusive, so I would suggest that you both stick to the rough guide of 200mg a day as a good all-round target. For women it makes particularly good sense, I think, to get into a good caffeine habit while you're trying to conceive, as current recommendations are to keep your intake low once you become pregnant.

Essential fatty acids

Read more on:
◆ Pages 17–18 & 95
▲ Page 62

Smoked mackerel pâté, page 217

As previously mentioned, oily fish are incredibly rich in one of the most beneficial types of fat: omega-3 fatty acid ◆. Although some studies have suggested that taking an omega oil supplement during pregnancy may offer certain benefits, such as helping to ensure the baby develops a healthy brain and nervous system, other studies suggest that taking a supplement could even improve your baby's intelligence. At the moment the evidence is not conclusive enough to make us think that we need anything more than a couple of 140g (5oz) portions of an oily fish such as salmon, trout, mackerel, herring, sardines, pilchards, kippers or fresh tuna each week. We can glean all the omega oils we need by eating this way – don't go over the two portions a week, as oily fish tends to store pollutant residues in their flesh, which we don't want to expose any unborn child to. If you've been taking supplements, it's best to stop as the Department of Health advises that pregnant women should avoid fish oil supplements during pregnancy because of their potentially high vitamin A content ▲.

If you're trying to get pregnant you should avoid eating shark, swordfish and marlin, and not eat too much tuna – no more than four medium cans or two fresh tuna steaks a week. This is because the mercury in these fish can potentially harm your unborn child's nervous system. All other fish are great for you, although as with the other oily fish, a couple of 140g (5oz) portions a week is the desired amount.

Folates and folic acid

Read
more on:
◆ Page 19
▲ Pages
58–63

It is now well recognised that folic acid ◆ also known as vitamin B9, is of critical importance both before and after conception in protecting your baby against neural tube defects. This is why we recommend that all women trying to get pregnant take 400mcg of folic acid each day, and continue right up until the end of the first trimester. Even if you fall pregnant unexpectedly, you should start taking the supplement straight away and continue to take it up until the end of the twelfth week. Our body doesn't absorb folic acid as well when it's in its natural folate form as it does when it's synthetic folic acid (this is one of those rarer occasions when the synthetic form outdoes the natural form), but it's good to eat foods rich in folate too as they are generally nourishing foods to include within the scheme of your diet. If you have a family history of neural tube defects you should discuss it with your doctor, who may recommend you take larger doses of folic acid.

Your pregnant body's needs

For some women, eating well while they're pregnant can be the easiest thing while others find foods they previously loved unpalatable and just crave starchy foods. They can therefore get into a bit of a muddle over how to balance what they know they should be eating with what will actually stay down and feel okay. Alternatively some women feel worried that their weight will spiral out of control so much that they'll end up feeling huge and not the person they want to be once they've given birth. Dieting while pregnant is not a good idea because it can compromise your baby's growth and development and also leave you feeling exhausted and depleted.

In this part of the book I want to take you through the key points of how best to balance your nutritional needs with those of your baby – which foods are best to focus on and which ones not to over-indulge in. Bear in mind that when you're pregnant you always need to have 'Is this safe for us to eat?' in the front of your mind ▲.

Nutritional supplements

You should avoid nutritional supplements other than folic acid unless an accredited clinical dietician has specifically prescribed them for you. This includes herbal remedies and some essential oils, as their stimulating effects on the body can be strong enough to cause problems – don't fall into the trap of thinking everything labelled natural and herbal is safe to take. Remember that opium, heroin and morphine can all be traced back to the poppy plant; and few would call these natural or safe!

Vitamin D

Read more on:
◆ Page 18
▲ Page 20

We've become more aware not only of how important vitamin D is for general health and bone strength ◆ but also of the significant problem in the northern hemisphere with women just not getting enough exposure to the sun's rays to manufacture vitamin D. Asian and Afro-Caribbean women living in cold climates are particularly at risk of having poor levels vitamin D, as dark skin is less efficient at manufacturing vitamin D from the sunlight. If you prevent your skin from being exposed to sunlight by covering up for religious or cultural reasons, your vitamin D levels can also be compromised. Low levels during pregnancy affect the growth and development of your baby, but you can ensure you both get enough vitamin D by taking a 10mcg (400 IU) supplement each day. You may also want to take a supplement while breastfeeding as we don't glean enough vitamin D from our diet to match our increased requirement whilst we're producing large volumes of milk.

Calcium

Although demands for calcium ▲ on the mother are high, during the latter stages of pregnancy your body will adapt through hormonal changes. You absorb more nutrients from your gut as a result of hormones such as oestrogen, lactogen and prolactin being present in your pregnant body, your body retains more of the calcium you absorb too – all this means that you don't need to take in more than the 700mg recommended for all women.

A well-balanced diet will give you all the calcium you need, however, you do need to pay particular attention to how much calcium you're including within your diet if you consume few or no dairy products, are vegan or have a poor vitamin D status (see above). Women who have a diet that is largely vegetarian and packed full of high-fibre foods, such as wholegrain, fruits and vegetables, can also hinder the absorption of calcium (despite the fact that these food are generally considered healthy). So it's this combination of factors which will require you to see whether you need to start including more non-dairy sources of calcium in your diet, the best ones being nuts, fortified soya milk and other soya products such as tofu (in moderation), dark green leafy vegetables and dried fruits. You may also benefit from taking a calcium supplement, although they are not usually very well absorbed.

A note about soya

There have been some concerns over the potential hormonal effects of eating a soya-rich diet when pregnant and whether or not it's a good idea to give a soya-based formula milk to a baby. The main concern seems to focus around the compounds known as phytoestrogens in soya and their effect on the development of the testicles. Animal studies have suggested that by mimicking oestrogen, these compounds could prevent the proper development of the reproductive system, causing a variety of problems later in life. But as these studies are based on rats and mice, it's difficult to assess what the result means for humans. Lots of mays and coulds, but I would suggest that if you're pregnant, avoid an overly soya-based diet. And when it comes to soya infant formula, you should only use it under the guidance of your doctor if your little one isn't able to tolerate any other infant formula.

If you're a young mum in your teens, since you're still growing and therefore have an increased need for calcium yourself, you may need to up your consumption of calcium-rich foods to cover what you both need – bear in mind that your baby will take from your calcium supplies first, and if you're not eating enough to meet what they need, as well as to ensure you're holding on to enough for yourself, you could end up with weak bones later in life. Dairy products are some of the best foods to include in your pregnancy diet, as not only do they contain the highest amounts of calcium but our bodies are able to absorb and use the calcium from these foods more easily than from non-dairy sources. If you can't take in dairy, for whatever reason, check out the alternative calcium-rich options mentioned above.

Iron deficiency

Bolognese sauce, page 210

Iron is one of the most essential nutrients for the growth and development of your baby and for enabling you to manufacture more red blood cells to support the pregnancy. We stop having periods and therefore don't lose any iron through menstruation, and get better at absorbing and mobilising our iron stores during pregnancy. Therefore it should be possible if you're eating an iron-rich diet when you're pregnant to meet the extra demand your pregnancy places on you. More and more women have low iron stores without knowing it. If you don't like eating much meat, whether you need to take an iron supplement will largely depend on your pre-pregnancy iron stores and how iron-rich your diet is throughout the pregnancy. The best way to check this is to keep in touch with your doctor so that they can run regular blood tests. If you find yourself suffering from any of the symptoms of iron deficiency anaemia, such as feeling depressed, overly tired, pale, breathless or losing your hair, your doctor may encourage you to start increasing the iron content of your diet or recommend a supplement. Iron deficiency anaemia can also make you more prone to infections and increase the risk of haemorrhage before or after the birth – when anaemia is severe it can hinder the development and growth of your baby. This shouldn't happen if you're in regular contact with your health team, are eating well and don't have any other underlying health problems that hinder iron absorption, such as coeliac or Crohn's disease. Occasionally in very severe cases you may need iron injections.

Feeling sick

This used to be referred to as morning sickness, which for many women is the time of day when it's at its worst. Some other women find themselves feeling continuously nauseous and off eating, which is a lot harder to manage. You've probably heard, and it's right in some cases, that the nausea is usually at its worst in the first trimester and for women who have undergone fertility treatments. Often you get changes in your senses too, which can put you off eating as your sense of smell can be heightened. Perfumes, smoke and the smells of certain foods can turn your stomach, which can be most frustrating if you're trying to eat a nourishing diet.

When you're feeling sick, try to get someone else to do as much of the food preparation as possible as it's often the cooking of foods that can make you feel queasy before you've even eaten a mouthful. Be aware that you need to be extra careful when reheating foods to ensure that they're well cooked and are not going to pose any food poisoning risk to you ◆. It's a great idea to get a willing friend or relative to stock up your freezer with some meals for moments when you're feeling below par. Another solution is to cook more than enough for a meal when you're not feeling sick, and in this way get ahead, as it takes no more effort to make enough pasta sauce for four meals as it does for one.

Read more on:
◆ *Pages 58–62*

There's really no rhyme nor reason to why morning sickness or indeed daily sickness makes you go off or crave certain foods, but one thing which does seem to help is to have a little something before you try to get moving in the morning such as plain biscuits or crackers.

The line on alcohol

The Government advises that when trying to conceive, women should give up alcohol altogether, while men shouldn't drink more than three to four units a day and should avoid binge drinking to prevent damaging the sperm. Although this is the official line, I think it seems horribly one-sided – perhaps it can be good for you both to take some time off the alcohol or at least cut your intake down. Being teetotal may not be what every couple wants or needs, as there is often anxiety within your relationship when trying to get pregnant. For example, you're both so desperate to succeed that having sex is dominated by thermometers, dates, positions, etc. In this case, a glass or two can lift the mood and make sex far more enjoyable. Make sure you've got some food in your stomach, if you don't want to fall asleep or feel woozy and therefore not in the mood.

The advice over whether or not it's safe to drink any alcohol while pregnant is hugely controversial. No one seems to agree and there doesn't seem to be objective data to give us a real steering on this. Some advise total abstinence, but the consensus seems to be that one to two units a couple of times a week is about the right level – it's always best to check for the latest advice. Bear in mind, though, that while so often we see one glass of wine given as a unit on the British alcoholic drinks tables, this refers to a pub measure (125ml/4oz) of wine, not the large glasses we tend to serve ourselves at home. One thing researchers do seem to agree on is that you can't store up your unused units and then have a whole bottle in an evening – binge drinking must be avoided at all costs.

Alcohol, like caffeine (and nicotine) passes from your blood into your breast milk. Whilst some research shows that alcohol can disrupt the release of two key hormones – oxytocin and prolactin – responsible for milk production, the odd glass of wine, beer or any alcohol is completely fine for you to drink, whilst breastfeeding. The old wives' tale of alcohol being good for milk production is nonsense. I find that the best way to enjoy alcohol is to feed your little one first, but at times, the odd glass can provide a much-needed respite before you start feeding.

Sometimes a more savoury style crispbread can do the trick – nibble a couple before you get out of bed. Ginger is also especially good at relieving nausea.

Not eating for a while can bring on nausea waves, so try eating little and often rather than going for just three main meals a day. This said, you need to watch that you don't just become a grazer and make sure you sit down to eat nourishing, well-balanced meals. Starchy foods seem to help stave off nausea more than protein-rich foods, so if you're having, say, a salad with chicken at lunchtime, put some crackers, bread or a small bowl of steamed rice with it and this could well settle your stomach. Many cultures consider rice to be one of the most settling of foods to eat when you're feeling sick. Try some cardamom-infused rice, which is not only delicious, but the slightly perfumed taste can help to settle your gut. Uncooked foods also seem to sit more comfortably and require less effort, but do make sure that you wash fresh fruit and vegetables well.

You may find that your whole body and eating clock goes through some weeks of turmoil. Play around with mealtimes and what you have in each meal too – eating a main meal at lunchtime may suit you better than in the evening. If you have a few days when you just can't stomach much, don't panic. The likelihood is that on other days, even if it's later on in the pregnancy, you will feel like eating something completely different. Remember that your baby will take exactly what they need from you, whether this is from what you've been eating that day or from your stores. A healthy diet will replenish your reserves and keep you in a good shape, so that when you've given birth you're not on your knees having been drained of all goodness.

Food cravings

Some women get the wildest of food cravings, which they feel they have to give in to – I don't have a problem with that as long as you try to build them into a structured and balanced diet. Enjoy the cravings, but don't mistake it for your body trying to tell you that you need more of something – there isn't any scientific proof that this is the case.

If you're craving very sweet, high-GI foods, watch their effect on your weight, as although there isn't any link between eating too much sugar and developing gestational diabetes (see below), it can be that you're gaining weight at a rate at which your body can't cope, specifically your pancreas. Very sweet foods, as is the case with high-fat foods, tend to be instantly gratifying but can leave you feeling pretty empty soon after. Try to incorporate cravings and preferences for specific foods into a well-structured plan rather than hoovering up an enormous tub of ice cream when watching TV, as delicious as it is!

Sometimes it's a craving for salt that hits the spot, in which case make sure that this isn't aggravating your blood pressure. Beware that salty foods can make you feel puffed up, making swollen ankles ten times worse.

Gestational diabetes

Gestational diabetes (GD) occurs in around 2 per cent of pregnancies and it usually crops up in the latter stages (most commonly in the third trimester). Your pancreas starts to struggle with the extra demands of a little person inside you so much so that it just can't maintain your blood sugar levels within the acceptable limits. Most women don't know they have it, as the symptoms of feeling more tired, etc. can be put down to being heavily pregnant, and it's usually not spotted until you have a urine or blood test. Gestational diabetes can usually be easily controlled by watching what, how much and when you eat. Occasionally insulin is needed, which requires a little more fine tuning (in which case you will also be referred to a dietician for specific help). More often than not, by watching that your diet is well-balanced, doesn't contain too many sweet foods like biscuits, cakes, sweet drinks, etc., and not too high in calories, you can keep blood sugar levels in check. Moderate exercise will help to maintain blood sugar levels too.

Constipation

Constipation is common in the latter stages of pregnancy when the baby presses on your internal organs and hormones slow down your bowel's ability to push food through. It can usually be relieved by upping your water intake and eating not only more of the higher-fibre foods such as wholegrain breads, cereals, pulses, nuts, fruits and vegetables ◆, but also specific fruits and juices such as prunes, figs and rhubarb. These can either be soaked, stewed or made into compôtes and will make a delicious start to your day, providing some much needed bowel-moving fibre, especially if served with Greek-style yoghurt and toasted nuts – scrumptious!

Read more on:
◆ Pages 30–32
▲ Pages 62–63

Raspberry baskets, page 246

Although it's not recommended to drink too much caffeine during pregnancy ▲, a hot cup of coffee or tea can act as a bowel stimulant, which could be just what you need to get things moving again. An alternative is to try hot water and fresh lemon, as there seems to be something about the warmth of the water that can get the body working.

Feeling uptight, stressed and exhausted can make constipation worse, and although it's far easier to write this than to put into practice, try to take your time in the bathroom – maybe have a warm bath, which will help to relax you before you try to go to the toilet. It's so often when you're rushing that constipation arises. Setting the alarm clock half an hour earlier in the morning is one idea, if this gives you time to be alone and peaceful in the bathroom before the madness of the day kicks in. Occasionally severe constipation can cause you to develop piles. If this becomes a real problem and monitoring your eating, drinking and relaxing doesn't seem to help, exercise can often make things easier. Exercise produces hormones that encourage the bowel to get moving as well as being a good stress reliever. It may work better if your hectic routine doesn't lend itself to yoga or relaxation – doing something you enjoy such as swimming could be just the constipation tonic you need. Some mums-to-be find that gentle massage and reflexology helps too.

Iron supplements can sometimes cause constipation, so talk to your doctor about changing to a different one, such as a herbal supplement if you suspect this. Don't take over-the-counter laxatives without consulting the doctor, as you need to ensure the remedy is safe for your baby.

Breastfeeding

There are countless nutritional reasons why breast is best, whether this is for just a few days or until your baby is ready to be weaned. These include: providing everything your baby needs to develop and thrive for the first six months, in the right amounts, at the right temperature and fresh; boosting your baby's immune system while their own is still developing – making them less likely to suffer from illnesses, such as diarrhoea, and vomiting, respiratory, ear and urinary tract infections, allergies, insulin-dependent diabetes, obesity and high blood pressure; it is also much cheaper than bottle-feeding. It is also a great opportunity for you to connect and bond with your baby though skin-to-skin contact. Breastfeeding also helps your womb to contract back to its normal size, and since milk draws on the fat stores laid down during pregnancy, it can help you lose your pregnancy weight. There are other advantages that will benefit your baby in the longer term – research has shown that breastfed babies are able to cope with stress later in life and interestingly, that they are more emotionally resilient if their parents divorce or separate.

However, as with all areas of parenting, you can only try your best, and if breastfeeding isn't possible or for you then this shouldn't mean disaster – there are perfectly good alternatives.

What should I be eating?

It may sound predictable, but a breastfeeding mother should eat a balanced diet with just a couple of tweaks. If you can eat well not only will you produce milk that's nourishing for your baby, but you will be far more likely to feel healthy yourself. Don't forget that your baby takes nutrients from you such as vitamins, minerals, fat, protein and carbohydrate.

Mums can find that they need to eat little and often or can feel ravenously hungry. So you may want to juggle your eating pattern to fit around these changes, such as having a larger breakfast or eating a cooked meal rather than a sandwich in the middle of the day. You need to make sure you eat a balance of things to produce good milk and leave enough nutrients for yourself. I would recommend that you eat an extra 300–400 calories per day for the first three months of breastfeeding and then an extra 400 calories a day, which equates to an extra good small meal, such as a cheese sandwich or a large banana and a couple of shortbread biscuits. Any more than that and you will find that your body holds onto the extra fat that was laid down during pregnancy and you won't be able to shift the weight.

When it comes to avoiding foods, the good news is that you can now eat those pregnancy no-nos, such as blue cheese. You do need to watch that you stick to just a couple of portions of oily fish each week, as you did during pregnancy ◆. Apart from the fish issue, there really aren't any hard rules, as everyone is different, but sometimes you may notice that your little one reacts badly after you've eaten certain foods. If they have more severe reactions to your milk, such as developing a skin rash or hives, have difficulty breathing, wheezing or congestion, or their stools turn green or mucousy, seek medical help.

Read more on:
◆ Page 63

Damson, pear & walnut muffins, page 253

I think that breastfeeding mums should drink about two and a half to three litres (10–13 cups) of water a day. This might sound a huge amount, but if you bear in mind that non-breastfeeding women should drink two and a half litres (10 cups) a day, it's not a lot extra for milk production. Some women feel completely fine, not drinking this much, but most end up feeling tired, ratty, headachy and constipated if they don't drink enough.

Feeling low

Being a new mum is exhausting and many women go through a period of 'baby blues' in the first few days after giving birth. There are various physiological and hormonal reasons for feeling down, while others just find that being responsible for a new life is overwhelming. Sadly, the difficulties in the first few weeks and months can lead to depression. You don't need to feel alone in this – ten to 15 per cent of new mothers suffer from post-natal depression, with many more experiencing weeks or months of intermittent feelings of low mood. Some women can even experience depression before giving birth.

I'm by no means saying that eating and food can cure what can be a very distressing and difficult time in a woman's life, but it's my experience as a mum that the types of foods you put inside your body can have an influence on how you feel emotionally, just as much as physically. We arrived home in the depths of winter and when my own mum, who had come with us to India to collect Maya, walked out of the door to go home, I was alone with a tiny, fragile, poorly baby. She was 15 months old but weighed under 4kg (9lb) and depended on me hugely to pull her through.

One of the first signs of depression is under or overeating, but by making sure you eat properly and resting as much as you can, the symptoms can become bearable. Sometimes medication is needed to treat the depression ◆, and although it is possible to breastfeed while taking some anti-depressants, some trigger side-effects such as weight gain. Some people get withdrawal symptoms when they stop taking them, which can compound how lousy you feel. In conjunction with your doctor's advice, looking at the types of foods and the way you're eating can enable you to help yourself through this tough time. So if you're feeling low, whether this be for a few days or something deeper and longer-lasting (in which case do seek some professional support), have a look at what you're eating, as food can be a great healer too.

Read more on:
◆ *Pages 45–49*

Chicken soup, page 231

Caring For Children

Much has been written about the nutritional needs of babies and toddlers, but there is a lot of confusing dietary information and you can feel anxious as a parent of a growing child. Weaning and the 'terrible twos' can be problematic, but it's vital that you establish good eating habits early in your child's life. For many parents, the time when their child starts going to school presents practical challenges: mornings become more rushed; school meals may be far from ideal, seldom offering what you'd like your child to eat; packed lunches can be time consuming to make and often come back hardly touched. All these issues are exacerbated by the fact that your child is that bit older, making them more opinionated about what they want and don't want to eat. At this age they're likely to be influenced by what their friends are eating, and perhaps one of the trickiest areas to navigate is how to withstand the pester-power antics from food manufacturers' marketing schemes.

Fortunately, I have a child who loves and appreciates food, likes to take an interest in how food is grown, prepared and shopped for (well, not all the time!). It has been, and continues to be, a glorious stage of my relationship with my seven-year-old daughter, but also a crucial one as good eating habits and an interest in food are instilled at an early age. I've chosen a few particular areas for discussion where I hope I can give reassurance and practical advice on how to move forward into your child's school-age.

Good eating habits

Read more on:
♦ Pages 98–99
▲ Page 14
● Pages 16–17

Roasted cherry tomato, basil & mozzarella pizza, page 239

There are times when children won't eat the food you put in front of them ♦, or you're pushed for time and have to grab something or cook something quickly that you know isn't ideal. But don't worry – children are much more resilient than we give them credit for, and ride the waves of coping with the odd not-great-eating day at times when you have to resort to this. Many children see fast and pre-packed food as a treat, so don't stress!

Three meals a day is the optimum eating routine, each containing something from every food group ▲. Even if your child isn't much of a breakfast eater, it's important that they eat something – they've had to tap into their nutrient reserves overnight, so their body needs a fresh supply of nourishment to get them through the morning. If they're off their main meals, don't sit there for hours waiting for them to give in (unless it's a trend) – give them a drink and something like a piece of toast and a banana to tide them over to the next meal.

It's not always easy, but the more you can eat together the better. Your children will see you eating similar foods and they love to copy and share. They will also see that the best way to eat is at a table concentrating on food and enjoying it – this is the perfect age to instil good habits.

Variety measured in handfuls

Use as wide a variety of foods as possible, to keep children's tastes diverse and also because each food has something unique about it. If you can introduce strong and varied flavours from an early age, there's less chance that you'll have a fussy child later on. If food is too samey and bland they'll develop conservative tastes.

A way to ensure that all the basic nutrient requirements are covered is to try to get into the habit of trying a different type of protein ● with each meal and a couple of different vegetables. There isn't any recommended number of portions of fresh fruit and veg for children per se, but I go for five a day (portions are smaller, though), the same amount that adults should be having.

Although variety is good, don't get hung up on having something different at every mealtime. Children can go through phases, and sometimes they will be in a bad mood, so just go for an easy option to avoid tempers getting more frayed; they're not going to start suffering from scurvy or some other vitamin deficiency disease if they don't have any fresh veg for a day – just try to get back into the swing of healthy eating as soon as you can.

Make the most of leftovers

Children don't need food that's freshly cooked from scratch every mealtime. Using yesterday's leftovers – for example bubble and squeak with an egg – can make a perfect tea. The only nutrients that aren't as plentiful in reheated and leftover food are vitamin C and folate. Fibre, proteins, energy, all the other vitamins and minerals are there in just as much abundance as they were in the first place, and if you want to increase the vitamin C level in a meal, for instance, serve it with some frozen or fresh vegetables – or simply have some fresh berries or other delicious fruit afterwards.

Start the day

Mornings can be chaotic, and it can be hard to get your child to sit down and eat breakfast, but the first meal of the day is one of the most, if not the most important of the day. Studies have repeatedly shown that children who eat breakfast have far higher vitamin, mineral and fibre intakes and are better nourished, which helps them to thrive in the classroom and enjoy playtime and sports.

For younger children, the best breakfast should be rich in slow-release energy, which can come from bread, muffins, crackers, cereal, porridge and fruit. The one thing that changes when children are a bit older is that their body is mature enough to cope with wholegrain versions of these carbohydrate-rich foods. When they're younger too much fibre can fill them up too quickly, compromise the absorption of minerals such as calcium and iron and prevent them getting enough energy from their diet ◆. Young children should be eating some of the less fibrous white breads, but from the age of 13 months they can eat the same as the rest of the family and tuck into wholegrain muffins, pitta breads and delicious mueslis and pastas.

Read more on:
◆ Page 94

Baked apples, page 240

Cereals can appear tempting, especially when you see the added vitamin and mineral flags, but they're seldom (especially the ones marketed at children) as healthy as they seem. They're often so full of sugar and salt that I just wouldn't touch the majority of them, apart from the odd treat. (I remember childhood holidays when we were allowed to choose from the selection of small boxes of children's cereals. Having my own little box to open contributed to the fun!) It's best to choose an unsweetened, simple wholewheat, oat- or bran-based cereal and then add fruit to make it sweet enough for your child's palate and for extra goodness.

You can get a large variety of types and quality of porridge oats – I used to hate them, but realised that when I made porridge using organic jumbo oats it had a great texture and natural nuttiness, as opposed to the mushy wallpaper paste a ground inferior oat turns into. Try toasting oat flakes in the oven or under the grill until they're golden brown, and add to porridge for a different taste and texture. If children are struggling with the larger oat flakes, just whiz them in a blender for a few seconds to make them smaller.

If you have the time and your child is up for a more substantial breakfast, there are a lot of benefits to be gleaned from including protein: protein not only gives the body a good hit of amino acids, but also slows down the absorption of the carbohydrate from the wholegrain, so that the energy you experience after eating, say, a boiled egg with your toast should be longer lasting.

There's a lot of nonsense written about eggs, which can make many parents restrict them in their child's diet, largely because they contain what has recently become a scare word – cholesterol. Yes, eggs do contain cholesterol, but the body is able to break it down, and they don't cause the bad sort of cholesterol to increase. In fact eggs are one of the most perfect foods for children (as long as there isn't an allergy issue) – they're versatile, easy to store, last a long time and can be boiled, scrambled, poached or fried within minutes. You could try beating them lightly with a dash of milk and dip slices of bread in to make scrumptious eggy bread – a good way to get reluctant egg-eaters to glean their goodness. Eggy bread is delicious with savoury toppings like sautéed mushrooms, lean ham, crispy pancetta, baked beans, grated cheese, tuna, or any oily fish like mashed sardines. Sardines tinned in tomato sauce are cheap, rich in omega-3 fatty acids and very more-ish when served on eggy bread, as is smoked trout or salmon, either on its own or with some cream cheese, or something vegetarian such as sliced tomatoes, grilled haloumi and cucumber or hummus … Virtually any topping works well with the light and yet satisfying eggy bread. Sweet toppings are delicious too – chopped fruit with a dollop of thick natural yoghurt, nut butter and banana is a Maya favourite.

Packed lunches

The reality is that despite recent school meals campaigns, many of our children's schools are reluctant to change their ways, or, as is the case with Maya's school, don't have a kitchen, making cooked meals out of the question. For whatever reason, thousands of children are either packed off with a lunchbox or given money to buy something on the way to school.

Children need a good lunch – the school day is long and the demands on their energy are great, whether it's a physically active day, or mentally draining. We know how it feels to be ravenously hungry – mood can dip, ability to concentrate goes out of the window – and our children are just as badly off, if not more so, since their early learning years require an enormous resilience in order to accumulate all the necessary life skills. If we put something into our stomachs that doesn't feel comfortable – too much, too salty, too sugary – our gut can start complaining, we get tummy aches, and if the food is too heavy all the body wants to do is sleep. We forget that our stomach is a muscle and needs oxygen to work. If you're running around, the oxygen may either be 'taken away' from the stomach, in which case you experience heavy, stitch-like discomfort, or the body's response to a big a meal is to release sleep-inducing hormones. School days sadly don't accommodate this luxury, so the trick is to put food in your child's lunchbox that is nourishing and sustaining enough to get them through the day but not too heavy to slow them down.

Read more on:
◆ Page 14
▲ Pages 90–91

Roasted tomato & couscous salad, page 218

Knowing where to start can be tricky, but as with all meals, the ideal is to include something from each food group ◆, as this replenishes energy stores, provides proteins for muscle strength, as well as vitamins, minerals and fibre. The solution is traditionally a sandwich, and this is what most parents find the easiest to put together. The bread choices we have today give us so many options, from traditional white and wholemeal sliced, to soft, crusty rolls, flat breads and dark rye-type pumpernickels ▲. The more you use your freezer, the more chance you have of making a bread-based lunch slightly more tantalising than the same old bread and filling. But this is not to say that a classic cheese or jam – I tend to use pure fruit spreads, or alternatively choose a jam with the highest fruit and lowest sugar content – sandwich should be frowned upon. You can freeze sandwiches if you wrap them well – just take a frozen pack out in the morning, and by lunchtime it will have thawed and be fresh-tasting. Fillings that do well frozen are charcuterie ham, jam (pure fruit spreads) or egg mayonnaise. Sometimes the sandwich can be a little on the soggy side, but children won't notice this, if you don't point it out – they're usually so ravenous and happy to have something inside their stomachs!

But there is life beyond the sandwich – crispbreads and crisp rolls are another option, as children like the crunchiness, and enjoy dipping crackers into a little pot of hummus or guacamole. I wrap the crispbreads in some foil to keep them dry and therefore crisp when they're opened The only thing you need to watch out for with crackers – which can be plain, wholemeal, seedy or those delicious Scandinavian crisp rolls – is that some of them can be rather salty, so check the label. Not only is too much

Read
more on:
◆ Page 44

Oxtail soup,
page 232

salt bad for anyone's health ◆, but it tends to make children thirsty, which could be a problem at school, depending on whether your child is lucky enough to be allowed access to water during the rest of the day. Crackers can work well with slices of charcuterie ham, roast chicken, cheese, etc., or, if your child isn't bothered by a slightly softer crispbread, can make a sort of sandwich with cream cheese, a soft cheese such as Camembert or a nut butter and sliced cucumber. Or they could be eaten alongside a flask of soup or a casserole from the night before. Dry foods can get stuck in children's teeth (crackers and crisps are the common culprits), so make sure they have a drink or eat some slippery fruit such as a few grapes or a satsuma, to wash them down.

Cold lunches can include pasta or rice salad, or couscous. Maya has recently got into potato salad, which is delicious in the summer when the potatoes are small, new and waxy, but also in winter, when even the older potatoes work well, as does combining them with sweet potato for another nutritious option (since it's a good source of beta-carotene). I make a simple new potato salad with a classic dressing, and use it as an easy way to make a good lunch out of not a lot of anything – a few added pieces of torn salami are delicious, as is something more exotic (there is no reason why children shouldn't like it) – smoked eel.

The great thing about thinking outside the traditional food box is that some foods, since they're not considered trendy, can be inexpensive, as producers know they can't let price be another barrier on top of unfamiliarity. The same can be said for cheaper cuts of meat such as ham hock, oxtail or offal – if your child enjoys eating liver, these make very nourishing casseroles or soups, that can be popped into a child's thermos flask for a hot lunch on a winter's day. They will also tide them over if you tend to find them ravenously hungry when you pick them up from school and you still have a long journey home or homework to finish before tea.

To snack or not to snack

Snacking is very different from nibbling or constant grazing, where your child consumes calories that don't register on the 'I've eaten' radar. A proper snack, which they eat when they can enjoy and concentrate on it, will keep them satiated for longer. The more you can help your child to be comfortable and okay with feeling hungry, the more able they will be to judge how much food they should be eating as they grow older. They are also less likely to struggle with excess weight and will have healthier teeth too.

Knowing when to give your child a snack depends on the situation and on your child – some days they won't be able to last from breakfast to lunch without a snack, while other days you'll be lucky to get just three meals into them, so snacks aren't necessary. It's best not to set yourself hard and fast rules, but have things with you in case it's one of those days when they need to eat more. Avoid getting into the routine of always giving them something between meals, as sometimes they don't need anything and the last thing you want is to fill them up on a snack so that they don't touch their main meals ◆. When they ask for food, check that they're not actually thirsty, as they can sometimes confuse their needs.

Read more on:
◆ Page 82
▲ Page 19
● Pages 110–113

Smoothies and juices

Smoothies and juices can be a great way to get children to take in a dose of vitamin C and folate ▲, along with some energising fruit sweetness which, if it's a no-added-sugar smoothie, can be better for them than one of the sugar-laden canned drinks. But, and it's a big but, I think we've become somewhat cajoled into believing that our children can drink an unlimited amount of these drinks. The latest claim from a well-known brand of smoothie, that each smoothie counts as two portions of the recommended five portions or fruits and veg a day, triggers some concerns for me. The notion that just one bottle can count towards two portions means you can become less resolved to get your child to eat more vegetables or pieces of fresh, unadulterated fruit, which have advantages over a smoothie because children have to chew them. This helps with speech development in younger children, which is a good thing.

Some smoothies can even give a child a sugar high, as they can drink quite a lot in a short space of time and there is a lot of fructose (natural fruit sugar) in them, which can aggravate mood and energy levels. The combination of a thick, sticky consistency, acids and sugars, albeit natural, in smoothies can lead to tooth decay.

No-added-sugar fruit squashes can be a useful and tasty addition if you want to make water a little different, but don't set a precedent for always giving your child squash from an early age. If you give them plain water as the norm and fruit squash as a treat, this stops them being so used to a sweet-tasting drinks. Be aware that several squash brands can contain additives and colourings, which in susceptible children can aggravate behaviour moods and energy levels and in extreme cases are linked to increasing the symptoms of attention deficit hyperactivity disorder (ADHD) ●. Cordials such as elderflower or ginger and lemon are very sweet, so again just use a dash every now and then.

Juices vary enormously and some juice connoisseurs say they can taste the difference, but nutritionally there is no difference between a juice made from concentrate, a chilled, freshly-made juice and one in a carton

My top snacks

If you can choose a snack with an intense flavour, such as a dried fig, your child will get that wonderful taste acknowledgement, rather in the way a few squares of 75 per cent or other good-quality chocolate will make you feel satiated. Snacks can be substantial, such as a small pot of pasta twirls with a couple of chunks of cheese, or a small filler such as an apple, a few grapes or a rice cake. Stock up on plastic containers of different sizes or save re-usable packaging and small plastic bags, washed well to store ready-to-eat snacks. It's worth buying a cooler bag and a flask that you can use for both keeping tap water cool and soup warm.

Snack ideas

- Fresh fruit or drained tinned fruit in natural juice, e.g. tangerines and chunks of pineapple.
- Dried fruits – ideally those without sulphur dioxide. Watch the ones with yoghurt coating, as they're often high in sugar.
- Raw vegetables, such as carrot, cucumber, celery, fennel, cherry tomatoes, etc. Serve with a little pot of hummus, bean dip, guacamole, tsatziki, or even make a dip from leftover cooked carrots and butternut squash blended with some natural yoghurt – whiz with a hand-held blender to the required consistency and serve with cucumber or celery sticks.

- Chunks of cheese or lean meat.
- Cottage cheese, with small rice cakes or grissini to dip.
- Wholemeal bread with wafer-thin ham, grated or cream cheese or nut butter – think beyond the peanut, as there are delicious hazelnut, Brazil and cashew nut butters too.
- Cooked cold pasta, drizzled with a little olive oil.
- Home-made soup – you can make it more substantial by adding pasta, beans, lentils etc.

stored on the shelf. I tend to go for blended apple mixes – I also use apple juice to sweeten cakes and biscuits and to soak muesli in overnight. Apple has one of the lowest GI values, which is a measure of how quickly a food gets absorbed and raises the blood sugar level, so it's my preferred juice for Maya too. The combination of fruit acids and fruit sugars can erode tooth enamel, which is why many dentists are encouraging parents to get their children to drink less juice. I'd suggest that a small glass of fresh juice, especially after a meal containing iron-rich foods each day is a good amount to aim for. Another option is to dilute fruit juice concentrate (available from health food shops and online).

Dairy foods

Read more on:
◆ Pages 16–21
▲ Pages 104–105

Tandoori chicken, page 213

Children of all ages can glean a lot of nourishment from dairy foods such as milk, yoghurt, cream, fromage frais and cheese. These foods provide the body with easily absorbed calcium as well as vitamins A and B12, plus protein and other vitamins and minerals, all of which are key for growth and healthy bodies ◆.

Whether you choose a full-fat or low-fat variety largely depends on how much fat you want your child to consume. The majority of the fat in dairy foods is saturated fat, and an excess of this can cause children (just as much as adults) to produce too much bad cholesterol, which can fur up arteries and increase the risk of heart disease. Cheeses, yoghurts and other types of dairy produce vary in the amount of saturated fat they contain, but it's not the best use of your brain power to go through their individual typical nutritional compositions – it also shouldn't be necessary with children to make a choice of cheese based on its fat or other nutrient content. I would suggest instead getting into some wise cheese-eating habits, as below, so you can enjoy the delicious upsides of cheese and not suffer from too many of the downsides.

Yoghurt

Yoghurt can be tricky – often packed with sugar, colourings and sweeteners – so my advice is to steer clear of the flavoured ones (even those with a misleading picture of fruit on the front). Go for the full-fat natural kind, either runny or the thicker Greek yoghurt, and add your own sweetness. This could be fruit compôte, stewed fruit, honey or nuts (not whole until your child is five), so at least you know what they're eating. Alternatively, you could make your own frozen yoghurt.

Use plain yoghurt in savoury dishes such as dips and soups and make a mayonnaise-style dip by using half natural yoghurt to half mayonnaise to give a lighter taste, or for coating chicken in a spicy masala yoghurt marinade. Better still, choose one containing live probiotic cultures ▲.

Milk

Once children are past the age of two – the recommended age when you can make the switch from full-fat (whole) (minimum 3.5 per cent fat) milk – one of the best ways to make sure they don't consume too much saturated fat is to change them over to semi-skimmed (about 1.7 per cent fat) or 2% milk. They will most likely be getting enough fat and calories from the rest of their diet, and the good news is that these lower-fat milks contain just as much calcium and actually, in the case of 1 per cent and skimmed (fat-free) (0.1–0.3 per cent fat, UK; less than 0.5%, US) milk, they do a touch better, containing slightly more calcium than full-fat milk. Taste-wise, semi-skimmed and 1 per cent milks are enjoyable and work well in sauces and other recipes, so it's an easy shift to make in the family's diet. Skimmed milk, in my opinion, is an acquired taste and doesn't work as well in cooking, since it lacks body when it's used in sauces, but it really depends what you're used to – if your child is a guzzler of milk and you're looking for a way to tweak their fat intake, 1 per cent milk may be the way to go.

Read more on: ◆ *Page 124*

Calcium is an essential nutrient for all children to help grow strong bones and reduce the risk of developing osteoporosis when they're older ◆. Many children don't receive the recommended daily intake of 500mg, which equates to 65g (2½oz) Cheddar cheese or 460ml (2 cups) milk.

There is no nutritional difference between ultra heat treated (UHT) milk and fresh milk – you get just as much protein, calcium, etc. So UHT milk can be a good option to use in cooking, especially as that way the slightly different taste isn't so noticeable. UHT milks are cheaper too, and since they're non-chilled products they last a long time – although when opened they need to be refrigerated in the same way as fresh milk.

There are subtle nutritional differences between the different dairy milks, such as goat's, sheep's and the classic cow's milk (sheep's milk is higher in calories than the other two, which are pretty similar). The fats in goat's milk are slightly different, which means that some children may find them easier to digest (they tend not to give them tummy aches), but this difference is so subtle that really the choice between whether you give your child cow's, goat's or sheep's milk should be down to preference. However, it is useful to know that the calcium, phosphorus, sodium, magnesium, zinc, and iron levels are higher in sheep's milk, which could influence your choice of milk. Bear in mind that the alternative dairy milks are more expensive than cow's milk, but essentially they all provide calcium and many other great nutrients such as B vitamins. When it comes to non-dairy milks the story changes, and there are huge differences that need to be considered. A word of warning when searching the Internet for information on non-dairy milks: remember that anyone can write an article and spout all sorts of pseudo-scientific rubbish, usually based around the simple notion that cow's milk is the devil's juice and you're 'poisoning' your children if you give it to them. This is nonsense, and unless your child has a genuine intolerance to cow's milk protein or lactose, or you're bringing them up vegan ◆, I would suggest using cow's milk as your main milk in their diet and using the other milks as variations in cakes, puddings, etc.

Read more on:
◆ Page 96

Soya milk

Soya milk is widely available in supermarkets and health food shops, and is increasingly being offered in cafés. There are many different varieties: sweetened, unsweetened, organic, fresh, long-life, vanilla-flavoured, mineral-enriched (such as calcium) and vitamin-enriched. Although you can also buy chocolate, strawberry, banana and other fruit-flavoured soya milks, be aware that these can be high in sugar – at least if you make your own you can control the amount of sweetness you add.

Some parents have real concerns about the presence of phytoestrogens in soya milk. These are oestrogen-like substances that occur naturally in many plants, including soya. There is some unease about the possibility that a large intake of phytoestrogens could have an adverse effect on a child's hormonal development, especially because children weigh much less than adults and the effect could therefore be potentially more pronounced. However, while studies on animals have shown that large amounts of phytoestrogens affect the development of reproductive organs and fertility, there is no evidence that there would be similar effects on people. So giving your child soya milk in the way that we typically use cow's milk, say a glass of milk a day, with perhaps a small pot of soya yoghurt and a meal based around soya protein, should be fine.

Too much of any food isn't good for us and it may be that in the future we will find out that too much soya milk isn't a good thing for children. So for this reason, if you're avoiding cow's milk for a health or medical reason, such as lactose intolerance, keep a variety of non-dairy milks in your child's diet – this way you'll be getting a spectrum of nutrients and minimising the potential health risks of too much of any one of them.

Rice and oat milks

Rice and oat milks contain far less protein, fat and calcium than cow's milk (depending on whether it's full-fat or semi-skimmed, of course). You can make up the difference in your child's diet with protein, fat, etc., but as far as calcium is concerned, the calcium even in the fortified versions of these milks isn't as well absorbed by the body as it is from cow's milk. If your child is following a dairy-free diet, seek advice from your doctor or dietician to see if you should be giving a calcium supplement. Rice milk is thinner and sweeter than soya milk and doesn't really work in hot drinks, but it's excellent on its own or with cereal. Delicious milkshakes and smoothies can be made by blending any milk alternative with fruit (either fresh or a dollop of pure fruit spread), good-quality chocolate powder or a non-dairy ice cream, for example one made with soya. Non-dairy milks vary in sweetness, as does fruit, so taste before you add anything sweet such as honey because it may not need much.

Nut and seed milks

Nut milks such as almond milk are available from health food stores, and make delicious smoothies, pancakes and puddings. But check out their nutrient labels, as they seldom provide as many minerals as dairy milks and have high fat and protein levels – though they can be useful if you're trying to boost your child's fat and protein intake and can be an essential part of a vegan or vegetarian diet ◆. Be aware, though, that children can be allergic to all kinds of nuts ▲, not just peanuts, so report any concerns you may have to your doctor immediately.

Read more on:
◆ Pages 92–96
▲ Pages 89–90

You can also make your own nut milks, and I particularly love almond milk. Hemp milk is a new addition to the non-dairy milk selection.

Tofu

Tofu is made by curdling fresh, hot soya milk, pressing it into a solid block and then cooling it – in much the same way that traditional dairy cheese is made by curdling and solidifying milk. It contains all eight essential amino acids and is a good source of protein. A staple ingredient in Thai and Chinese cookery, it can be cooked in different ways to change its texture from smooth and soft to crisp and crunchy.

Try slicing, marinating and grilling it, or chopping it into smallish pieces and frying it with garlic until golden. Sliced raw tofu can be used instead of mozzarella in the classic Italian salad with tomato and avocado. Silken tofu is a creamy, softer product that works well in puréed or blended dishes such as flans and quiches, and is ideal for making puddings such as mousses. It's better to give children the silken kind rather than the pre-marinated kind as it tends to be less salty, but as long as you're not using salt elsewhere either variety should be fine.

Cheese

- Grate cheese for sandwiches rather than slicing. Grating increases the surface area and makes your taste buds tingle more from a smaller amount of cheese.

- If you're after an intense flavour, use a cheese that has been matured for longer. There are many different varieties – try them in dishes such as cauliflower cheese – blue-veined cheeses are delicious. The advantage of a strong-tasting mature cheese is that you need a smaller amount than you would using a milder one to get the same cheesy flavour. This means you consume less saturated fat, you need less salt when you're flavouring the dish and the piece of cheese will last longer.

- Use a little mustard, either powder or creamed, to bring out the cheese flavour in sauces, soufflés and pies.

- Although chunks of cheese make a nourishing snack, it's a good idea to have something alongside them such as grapes, pieces of apple, crackers or grissini. Not only does this provide some bulk, sustaining your child for longer, but having a couple of different textures and tastes also stimulates the part of the brain that acknowledges satiety.

- If you make your child a cheese sandwich, try to incorporate something rich in fibre such as wholegrain bread, or have an apple with it. If the child also has a drink of water, the fibre in the bread or the apple will swell and stimulate stretch receptors in the stomach that send signals to the appetite centre and make them feel satisfied.

- When slicing cheese, use a cheese slicer, as this gets you out of the habit of cutting unnecessarily thick pieces.

- I'd much rather give Maya a smaller amount of a higher-fat cheese that she'll enjoy than go for a disappointing half-fat or reduced-fat cheese. However, if your child is gaining too much weight, and you have got into the good habits above but are still looking for ways to reduce calories, try some of the reduced-fat varieties available.

- Cut the rind off soft rind cheeses like Brie and Camembert – this reduces the fat content. When you serve these soft cheeses, and also cheeses without rinds, which include sheep's and goat's cheeses, you shouldn't need any butter.

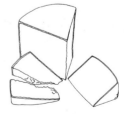

Fats

Read
more on:
◆ Pages
17–18
▲ Pages
94–95

Roast mackerel
with potatoes
& thyme,
page 215
Cashew nut
butter,
page 229

While your child needs some fat to grow and develop, too much of any sort of fat can lead to heart disease ◆. There are many healthier alternatives, so favour the Mediterranean fats as a rule. It isn't good to deep-fry everything, but there's nothing wrong with a drizzle of vinaigrette dressing on a salad, or new potatoes with a small amount of butter. It's all about moderation.

Ideally everyone should have a couple of 140g (5oz) portions of omega-rich oily fish each week. Girls and women of child-bearing age should stick to two portions (because of concerns over the build-up of toxins in the body, which could harm babies born to them in the future), but boys and everyone else can have up to four portions a week. With recent concerns over the mercury levels in tuna, however, I wouldn't go above a couple of portions of tuna a week for either boys or girls. If you don't like fish, or if you'd like non-fish sources, turn to oils such as hemp and linseed (flaxseed), walnuts and their oil, and seeds such as sunflower and pumpkin. I grind the seeds up to improve absorption and use them in porridge, smoothies, breakfast cereals, crumbles and cakes.

Butter and margarine

Butter and olive- or vegetable-based spreads are good choices. Check the labels to ensure they don't contain hydrogenated fat, as this can lead to trans fats, the unhealthiest sort of fat – although most manufacturers have thankfully removed these from spreads. While too much saturated animal fat isn't the healthiest (it can increase the risk of heart disease), there is nothing wrong with a spread of butter in moderation. One way to keep your salt intake down is to use unsalted butter.

Nut butters

Nut butters provide a delicious, sustaining spread. They are a great source of protein and 'good' mono-unsaturated fats. They also contain fibre and minerals such as zinc. There are so many different ones available, however you can make your own – which I like to do, as you can control what you put in them.

Choosing and using oils

There are so many deliciously healthy oils – rapeseed, hemp, avocado, nut oils – available in supermarkets and they provide a good source of energy ▲. Rapeseed oil, like hemp oil, contains very useful omega-3 fatty acids. Hemp oil varies in its taste and is sometimes a touch strong, so try different brands until you find the one you like best – I favour oils that are lighter on the palate. I love to use avocado or nut oils in dressings and for drizzling over grilled vegetables, sesame seed oil is my chosen oil for stir-fries.

I think it's a shame to use extra virgin and other more boutique oils for simple frying. I tend to use a non-virgin olive oil or a vegetable oil for frying onions, garlic, vegetables, etc. as a base, and then, if the final dish needs a drizzle of something more flavour-enhancing, bring out the bottle of special oil. As well as not wanting the oil to be too hot, you don't want it too cool. Food will soak up oil that's too cool, and therefore the fat and calorie content will be much higher than if the oil is hot enough to make the food sizzle when you pop it into the pan – hot oil quickly seals the food and this stops the fat being soaked up. One test is to drop a piece of bread into the hot oil – if it sizzles and bubbles within a few seconds, the temperature is about right. Bear in mind that nut and other vegetable oils have different burning and smoking points, so try them out to see how they react on your cooker and in your pans. Burnt oils often turn bitter, and oils are more likely to produce trans fats when they get too hot, which aren't good for us – this doesn't usually happen with oils if they're only overheated once, but try not to overheat oils at all. When using oil for deep-frying, use fresh oil if possible, although it's fine to reuse it a few times.

Nuts

Nuts are good to have in your storecupboard. Peanuts are in fact legumes, as in they grow beneath the ground, unlike other proper nuts, such as walnuts and hazelnuts. Whole nuts shouldn't be given to very young children, but once over the age of five, your child should be able to manage them without choking. Ground nuts and nut butters are good to include in your family's diet from an early age (as long as there is no allergy issue).

More-ish nutty biscuits, page 248

Crushed nuts can be added to yoghurt to provide a little more nourishment – the crunch factor can be fun too, especially if you make up a bowl of mixed crushed nuts and dried fruits that children can 'tip' or dip their hand into, a far healthier version of the manufactured tippy-style yoghurts that children seem to love.

You can eat nuts straight from the pack, but also try toasting them lightly first to maximise crunch and excite the highly flavoured volatile oils, either in a dry pan or the oven (eight to ten minutes at 180°C/ 350°F/gas mark 4 will do it; you don't want them black, just tinged here and there with golden brown). Throw a few of your toasted nuts over salad leaves dressed with a little nut oil and lemon juice, and toss with crisply sizzled shreds of leftover meat such as roast chicken. Make them into a quick lunch by tossing them with roasted vegetables, crumbled goat's cheese and rocket, or stir into bulgur wheat with lots of chopped mint and cubes of hard goat's cheese or mature Cheddar.

Carbohydrates

Read
more on:
◆ Pages
30–32
▲ Page 94
● Pages
84–86

Wholemeal
soda bread,
page 237

Children need a source of carbohydrate-rich food in each meal. Porridge and wholemeal food all provide a good source of energy as well as fibre ◆. Wholemeal is good news for all the family, although too much fibre is not always a wonder food for young children ▲. To give you an idea, my rule of thumb is, that children over two and a half years old have two-thirds of their bread, pasta, etc. as wholemeal and the remaining third as white. Some children manage to get enough energy and thrive on an entirely wholemeal diet, so it's just a matter of seeing how your little one responds to wholegrain goodness.

Make porridge with semi-skimmed or full-fat milk ● as children need some fat to provide enough energy to grow and to absorb essential vitamins. Try topping porridge with berries (which can be frozen), apple purée, chopped fruit, dried fruits, half a teaspoon of pure fruit spread, a dollop of stewed fruit or a drizzle of honey for a delicious, sweet taste with just a small amount of sugar. The glycaemic index (GI) of honey is slightly lower than granulated sugar, so this breakfast keeps children satiated for longer. Pure fruit spreads and no-added-sugar jams have a more intense fruity taste and don't contain refined sugars, which, I think, is better for everyone.

Bread

There's nothing wrong with white bread (it gives children energy and some extra calcium, iron and B vitamins such as folic acid, since the flour is fortified), but if you can, choose a half and half loaf, which contains slightly more fibre. There are lots of different types of wholemeal bread on the market, from the lighter, fluffy wholemeal bread to the denser, seedy, German-style wholemeal, so try a few until you find one every member of your family enjoys.

If your child isn't gaining as much weight as they should, or if they're unable to finish a meal and have an upset tummy, switch to breads with slightly less fibre – brown, granary or a half and half loaf. Breads like ciabatta and focaccia contain olive oil, are delicious, and are good for them, especially if they have a small appetite – a mouthful contains more calories than wholegrain (because of the oil) and can tempt a little one's jaded palate, although these breads are usually based around white flour, so contain less fibre.

Making bread by hand also means that you can fill it with all sorts of things, from fruit purées, seeds and nuts, to savoury tapenades, and mould it into whatever shape you fancy – you also know exactly what's going into it. You can add almost anything to the bread mixture to make it unique – olives, olive oil, herbs, dried fruits or nuts – or make a brioche-style loaf using milk as a base in which to warm the yeast. Alternatively, for people who can't tolerate dairy produce, use fruit purées or apple juice.

Quinoa

Quinoa (pronounced keen-wah) is an ancient sesame-seed-sized kernel, which we think of and treat as a grain, although technically it's not (it's the seed of the goosefoot plant). Quinoa is a good source of carbohydrate, protein and fibre, and also contains B vitamins and a little polyunsaturated fat. It's gluten-free, so it's useful for children who have problems digesting gluten. You can buy quinoa flour in supermarkets, health food shops and online, to make pancakes, bread and cakes.

The seeds are usually eaten cooked, like rice (although you can sprout them too, see below), but you need to wash them well first, to get rid of any residue that may leave a bitter taste. Cook quinoa for about 15 minutes for a rice-like texture. You can add the uncooked seeds to soups and casseroles (as long as there's plenty of liquid for them to absorb), and you can make them into porridge, just the same as with oats, using water or milk. You can roast the seeds in a non-stick frying pan for a few minutes first if you like, until you get a waft of nuttiness. The toasted seeds will keep in an airtight jar in a cool place for weeks.

To sprout quinoa, soak two tablespoons of seeds in a jar of cold water for two to four hours, then drain and rinse twice a day for two to four days. Sprouts will quickly appear and are delicious in salads or stir-fries.

Vegetarianism

Whether or not you're going to include meat in your child's diet may be your own choice or may come from your child. Life is easier if you can make one meal for the whole family rather than having to come up with both a meat and a veggie option, but try not to make a big issue of it – you could always cook a lamb chop or roast a chicken for the non-vegetarians to have alongside a vegetarian dish.

It's perfectly possible for children to thrive as vegetarians and in fact there are some real plus points, since studies have shown that vegetarian children consume more fresh fruits and vegetables and are therefore less likely to suffer from obesity, bowel cancer and heart disease when they are adults. Nowadays there are many recipes and diverse ingredients available, not just at specialist food retailers and online companies but even in supermarkets.

However, you do need to watch a few areas of your child's diet to ensure that they're getting the key nutrients in plentiful quantities. Some people call their children vegetarian when in fact they eat fish and seafood – technically this isn't what being a vegetarian is about. The majority of vegetarians still include dairy and eggs, which makes things

Protein for vegetarians

Legumes: Chickpeas, butter beans, black-eyed beans, kidney beans, borlotti beans, haricot beans (used for baked beans)

Pulses (dried legumes): Lentils, split peas, dried green peas

Soya products: Miso (fermented soya bean paste), tofu (soya bean curd), tempeh (soya meat alternative), tamari (wheat-free soy sauce)

Nuts: Almonds, peanuts, cashew nuts, Brazil nuts, walnuts, hazelnuts, pine nuts, nut milks

Seeds: Sesame seeds, sunflower seeds, pumpkin seeds, linseeds (flaxseeds), quinoa

a lot easier as it gives a larger spectrum of foods to choose from (dairy and eggs are excellent sources of protein and key nutrients).

Protein

Read more on:
◆ Pages 16–17
▲ Page 20
● Pages 19–20

The first essential nutrient to be included in plentiful supplies is protein, which children need to build and replenish a strong digestive, muscular, hormonal and immune system ◆. Animal protein is what we call complete as it contains all the essential amino acids, but unfortunately the same can't be said about vegetable protein, with the exception of soya (and soya products such as tofu) and seaweed. It's simple to get around this by eating a wide variety of plant-based proteins – if you look at the list below you will see there are plenty of delicious foods to choose from.

Vitamins and minerals

If children are eating a varied vegetarian diet containing a plentiful supply of different proteins, cereals, vegetables, fruits and some dairy they should be getting a good balance of essential vitamins and minerals. But calcium, iron and vitamin B12 deserve special mention when you're vegetarian as they can often be lacking.

Calcium is essential for bones and teeth, and is also needed to help muscles work properly ▲. It is much easier to ensure that children take in enough calcium if they eat dairy produce. There is far less calcium in non-dairy foods, so if dairy isn't on the menu every day, discuss the issue of your child taking a calcium supplement to help ensure they're reaching their requirement.

The most easily absorbed sources of iron are liver and lean red meat, but for vegetarians some iron can be found in egg yolks, peaches, apricots, figs, nuts, bananas, green leafy vegetables, seaweed, watercress, avocados, fresh herbs (particularly parsley), pot barley, baked beans in tomato sauce (always a good standby), nuts, oatmeal, lentils, sunflower seeds, fortified breakfast cereals, wholemeal bread and brown rice. Unfortunately, however, unlike meat sources, vegetarian sources of iron need a helping hand from vitamin C to be absorbed. The secret is to eat vitamin C-rich foods in the same meal as the iron-rich ones – this means getting into the habit of serving iron-rich vegetables followed by a portion of fresh or tinned-in-juice fruit. All fruits contain vitamin C but some are richer than others: kiwis, strawberries, blueberries, blackcurrants, papaya, oranges and mangoes.

Vitamin B12 ● is found in almost all foods of animal origin, but vegetarians can also find it in yeast extract, fortified breakfast cereals, seaweed and spirulina. Dietary deficiency of vitamin B12 is rare in younger people and only occurs among strict vegans. B vitamins particularly vitamin B12, are often low in the vegan diet. You can buy fortified cereals, soya drinks, spirulina (a form of algae available in capsule or powder form, which you can stir into smoothies) and low-salt yeast spreads (the full-blown ones are far too high in salt for kids). However, it's not easy to get children to eat enough of these foods to cover their basic requirement, so consider giving them a supplement containing 1.2mcg per day until they're nine years old and then increase this to 1.8mcg per day.

Fibre

In general we all need to eat more fibre – a high-fibre diet is satisfying, since fibre helps keep us satiated, reduces the risk of heart disease and many cancers, and helps to keep our day-to-day gut movements healthy and regular. But with children, especially vegetarian children, you need to ensure they're eating enough but not too much. Too little fibre can cause constipation, which is miserable for children ◆, but on the other hand too much can lead to your child becoming listless, low in energy and (especially common in vegetarian children) anaemic. This is because too much bulk from fibrous foods and too many phytates, which bran and other wholegrain cereals contain, inhibit the absorption of iron.

Read more on:
◆ *Pages 106–108*

Butternut squash & red lentil dahl, page 204

Vegetarian children are more susceptible to this scenario simply because a vegetarian diet naturally tends to focus on vegetables and fruits. Parents who choose to be vegetarian can be great vegetable cooks and lovers of all food healthy and wholegrain, so before too long, if vegetables and bulky wholegrains are too large a part of a young child's diet, their body can be overloaded with fibre. Note also that too much fibrous food without enough water can in itself cause constipation, so children need to have a good couple of glasses of water with a meal in order to provide enough fluid to enable the fibre to work for rather, than against, keeping the gut regular.

Watch out for your child's weight not increasing as it should, or you might notice that they are more tired and grumpy than usual. Any of these signs could indicate too much fibre in their diet.

Getting the energy levels right

Children, especially vegetarian children, need good healthy sources of energy in their diet, which they usually glean from fats and carbohydrates. There are two main types of fat: those that come from animal foods such as butter, cream, cheese, yoghurt and milk, and those that come from vegetables, seeds, nuts, olives, avocados and oils, such as rapeseed, hemp, sunflower and safflower oils. I like to base much of my diet around vegetarian sources of fat for two reasons: first, cakes, muffins, biscuits, sauces, etc. are delicious when made with nut milks, or oils such as rapeseed or hemp, nut butters, seeds and other energy-rich ingredients. Second, vegetable fats largely (with coconut oil being one notable exception) consist of unsaturated fats such as monounsaturated fats – some of the healthiest types of fat for our hearts ◆.

Read more on:
◆ Page 17
▲ Pages 17–18

This isn't to say that animal fats are bad for children – there are great advantages for including dairy foods in a vegetarian diet. They are great energy-giving foods and also provide calcium and vitamin D.
You just need to watch that vegetarian children don't have their diet dominated by too much dairy (an easy trap to fall into, since dairy foods can be pretty more-ish and provide an easy and practical option) – a diet too rich in dairy can be higher in calories than even a young, growing child needs, racking up their saturated fat intake, which their cardiovascular system won't appreciate.

Although soya milk and soya products contain plenty of protein, they tend to be very low in fat, so they're good for children's hearts but are not great for boosting energy. Include other vegetable fats too – for example, you could make porridge made with soya milk but then stir in a dollop of nut butter or a teaspoon of ground seeds and nuts.

Omega-3 fatty acids

Omega-3 fatty acids are hard to find if you follow either a vegetarian or a vegan diet. The main dietary source of omega-3 will be from ALA ▲, unfortunately, due to the body's inefficiency at converting ALA to EPA and DHA, it's hard to provide these two vital fatty acids in the amounts the body needs. You'd have to really be tucking into lots of plant sources of ALA, which isn't that practical, so I'd suggest giving your child a vegetarian omega-3 supplement just to cover their needs. This will take the pressure off, and means you can enjoy using seeds, nuts, etc. as part of their general diet without thinking they've got to consume a certain amount in order to meet their omega-3 requirement. It's not easy getting a vegan diet right for your child, so do as much research as you can, and ask your doctor to refer you to a paediatric dietician who can assess and advise you on the overall nutrient levels of your child's diet.

Vegetarian ready-made foods

We all need a helping hand now and again, so having a stock of ready-made frozen foods such as vegetarian sausages and burgers can be a life-saver when you need to put together a quick and easy meal.

But don't assume that the word 'vegetarian' on the label or the lack of meat means they're full of healthy ingredients – you would be shocked to see that fat, sugar, additive and salt levels can be high (in some cases far greater than the non-vegetarian options). So check the labels and try to balance a high value with something nutritious alongside.

The vegan diet

It's a lot easier to follow a vegan diet now that supermarkets, health food shops and online suppliers stock such a wide variety of non-animal dairy produce and ready-made vegan meals. Feeding a vegan child can be a little daunting, as you need to avoid all animal produce, so here are a few of my storecupboard favourites.

- Seed pastes like tahini can be stirred into bean salads and is the basis of hummus (a staple in our house). Tahini can be spread on bread or crackers as a butter substitute, stirred into a bowl of pasta or used to top jacket potatoes.
- My favourite – nut butters such as peanut, cashew, hazelnut and almond. They are yummy on bread and rice cakes and good in vegetable casseroles and bakes. Whole nuts should be avoided until your child is over the age of five.
- Vegetable oils – check out rapeseed, avocado, nut and hemp oil – can not only give a different taste to recipes but also contain different fatty acids, for example walnut oil is rich in omega-3 fatty acids and avocado oil is rich in monounsaturated fats. Too much fat isn't good for any child, but since the vegan diet is generally very bulky, it's important you don't shy away from using oil or something rich in each meal. Vegan children need the calories and energy hit that fats bring, so drizzle oils over vegetables, dip bread in oil at the table, make a sandwich with creamy hummus and roasted vegetables or top warm toast with tahini and sliced peaches. Try to buy speciality breads made with olive oil, such as focaccia, or make your own, as they're higher in fat and more energy-rich than standard breads.

- Avocados are wonderfully creamy and rich in fat – good on jacket potatoes, in salads and sandwiches, even mashed on rice cakes spread with nut butter and sliced banana.

Cooking the slow way

It's all very well and good throwing something to eat together at the end of the day, but one of the ways I juggle being a working mum is to rethink the food preparation routine so that we can walk through the door and know that all we have to do is find a plate. Slow cooking works especially well for me, as I'm an early riser – I can prepare the meal before Maya wakes up and still have time at the end of the day, when we're both tired, to concentrate on getting through homework knowing that tea is taken care of.

If you want to shift your own routine around, either get up earlier, or, if you're more of a night owl, prepare your evening meal the night before. Think about investing in a slow cooker – they're electric and are built with safety sensors so that they can be left for hours to gently cook the food. (You can set them to come on automatically so that the casserole's cooked by the time you get home.) Alternatively, if you're an Aga enthusiast, find the right sort of cooking pot to allow the casserole to simmer away all day in the slow oven.

There are many nutritional advantages to letting foods cook slowly. First, if you give ingredients time to simmer, mix and infuse, the natural flavours will develop and deepen, so you should need less salt at the end (get used to tasting your food just before you serve to prevent adding salt from force of habit). Try using black pepper first to see whether that tweaks the flavours sufficiently and maybe a squeeze of fresh lemon too. Using garlic, and intense herbs like bay and sage, are my favourite ways to provide big flavours without using much salt. Casseroles and tagines work well if you add some wine before cooking, as it enhances the flavours but the alcohol evaporates, so the calorie and alcoholic impact is nil. Remember to use only wines you'd be prepared to drink and don't just bung in any old past-it plonk!

Slow cooking means that vegetables and pulses such as beans and lentils are well cooked making them easy to digest. It also means that less confident cooks can use root vegetables such as celeriac, swede and parsnips, without having to worry about the exact timing – just throw it all in and let the casserole do the work for you. I always love mushy vegetables in sauces, and children with sensitive guts ◆ find them easily digestible. They absorb more antioxidants from a cooked carrot than they would from a raw one, which may upset their gut and pass through before they've had a chance to properly digest and absorb all the goodness from it. One-pots are fantastic for children who don't like the look of vegetables in their crisp state – you can trick them into eating a meaty casserole

Read more on:
◆ Pages 108–110

Chicken, tomato & sausage hot pot, page 202

knowing that there are four or five vegetables in the sauce. You can even liquidise the sauce if they're particularly fussy eaters, add extra stock and blend everything to make a hearty soup. While heat (especially over a long time) destroys a lot of the vitamins B and C, within a casserole you keep all the cooking liquid that the water-soluble vitamins such as vitamin C leach into, so you'll still get some nutrients from the sauce.

Cooking slowly allows you to choose more economical cuts of meat such as knuckles, hocks, oxtail, brisket, and also use pheasant and other game, which need slow cooking to tenderise the flesh. If you're worried about the higher fat content of cheaper cuts, first think about what you're going to serve them with – maybe jacket potatoes, a quick-soak couscous, or a hunk of fresh wholegrain bread. You can reduce the fat content by using the sauce from the casserole instead of butter or oil on these accompaniments: stir it into couscous instead of adding oil, or use bread to mop up the juices instead of spreading it with thick lashings of butter. If you have time to let the casserole cool down, you may like to skim the fat off the top, either with one of the fancy brushes or pipettes you can buy, or just by lifting the fat off if it's gone solid. But remember that, in spite of the huge anti-fat lobby that's so prevalent in our society, we – especially children – need some fat in our diet for flavour and to help our bodies absorb fat-soluble vitamins ◆. No one can convince me that eating a home-cooked casserole containing good fresh ingredients including high-fibre vegetables, beans or lentils is anything other than great for my family's health.

Read more on:
◆ *Pages 18–19*

Fussy eating

Food tantrums can break any parent's resolve. Maybe it would help if we just ditched the notion that mealtimes should be relaxed and without any emotional outbursts, whether from you or your child, and regard anything other than complete meltdown as a positively great mealtime! Joking aside, until you've been a parent and experienced how food and emotions can be so entwined, it's impossible to know how tough it can be to get right. I could write a whole book on how parents need to lead the way with instilling good eating habits, but what may work on one occasion and for one child may not work with the next. What I do know, from helping many parents with fussy eaters, is that the sooner you can instil the idea that you eat what you're given the better. Modern lives where children eat separately from their parents, and the concept of 'meals for one' or 'children's meals', imply that everyone can in theory have something different to eat. What we have created is a nation of very fussy eaters who have been allowed to dictate what they fancy eating. It's hard as a parent when you're shattered and want to avoid conflict at mealtimes, but beware of giving in when toddlers try to manipulate what they eat.

It's ideal if you can either sit and eat the same food with your children, or at least cook one pot of food so that they know this is all that's on offer. Okay, children will have preferences, and there will be foods that they're less keen on, but stick to your guns and reward them for trying even a small mouthful of the food – say with a sticker chart. Although getting into the habit of rewarding them with a chocolate or something sweet they love isn't ideal, don't feel bad if you sometimes resort to this.

Not cooking them something else when they refuse to eat is a really tough thing to do. You may well fear that they'll end up ravenously hungry or wake up in the night, and of course there will be times when you can let the bar down, but it's generally best to stick with the policy that you eat what you're given and don't get anything else. Hungry children will eat eventually, and they'll soon start to change when they know their fussy eating requests don't get much of a reaction. Obviously try to choose something they will enjoy, and see some wins on their sticker chart at the next mealtime if you can, but if they start playing up and saying they no longer like this, then you know it's a behavioural rather than a taste issue. To test whether they truly dislike something or are just being difficult, I'd suggest trying each new food eight or ten times before putting it to one side for a few weeks – at which point try it again and see if the sticker chart motivates them then. Just because they didn't like it before doesn't mean it won't prove a hit in a few weeks' time. The more calm and clear you are that they will only get what's been cooked, the sooner they will respond – but it takes the patience of a saint!

Tired all the time?

Read more on:
◆ Page 11

My mum's chicken pie, page 211

If you've noticed your child is below par and lacks go-getting energy, there may be a simple solution or you may need to do a bit more investigating, such as keeping a food diary ◆ to check that they're getting a varied diet of nourishing foods.

Check they're getting enough exercise, as lack of fresh air and running around can make them feel tired. I find when Maya's over-tired the best thing is a walk or cycle ride as the exercise produces endorphins which lift her mood and increases her metabolism, making her physically tired enough to go to sleep as soon as she hits the pillow. Lack of sleep is an obvious cause, but maybe you could do things differently in the evening to help them nod off – TV last thing before they go to bed could be causing dreams or stopping them getting off to sleep early, while a bath followed by a story and a few drops of lavender oil on the pillow usually works a treat.

Tiredness can be a key symptom of dehydration. Many little ones don't drink enough water – it's especially easy to become dehydrated when the weather's hot or if they're been especially active. They also need more water if they've eaten a salty snack such as a packet of crisps.

Anaemia (the lack of haemoglobin, which carries oxygen in the blood around the body so that our cells can use it to produce energy) causes children to be constantly tired, pale, possibly headachey, with lots of crying. See your doctor who can diagnose anaemia with a blood test. It's usually caused by too little iron in the diet, so focus on boosting their intake of iron-rich foods ◆.

Read more on:
◆ *Page 20*

Too much fibre can prevent children from getting enough energy in their diet. It's hard to give exact guidelines, as some children can glean enough energy when they're eating wholemeal all the time but others may need a break from the wholegrains. Try more white pasta and bread to see if it makes a difference.

Surviving tantrums

While it's perfectly normal for young children to lose it occasionally, there's losing it in a small and containable way, and then there's those dreaded meltdowns which often happen when it's the last thing you need. I've found that what children eat and drink, and when they do it, can have an impact on lessening the severity of the meltdowns.

Make sure they're drinking enough water, as a dehydrated child is far more likely to be a moody one. About one to one and a half litres (4–6 cups) of water a day is a good target to aim for, but remember, when they're having a meltdown they often get hot and sweaty, so they lose more fluid. If water doesn't interest them, try adding a small amount of apple juice, as this can feel like a real treat and since apple juice has one of the lowest GI values it's less likely to aggravate blood sugar levels – which I find can be a precipitating factor in tantrums.

Try to get children to eat regularly. Sometimes we're caught out and schedules go wrong, and this can be one of the reasons why they're more likely to get out of control – they just haven't had enough food to keep their blood sugar at the best level and this can affect mood. When you know it's going to be a stressful or important day, try to think ahead as much as you can to ensure mealtimes are regular. I find a big breakfast with eggs, grilled sausages and wholemeal toast sets us off on a good footing. If you're already mid-meltdown, cajole them into having something to eat if you suspect that lack of nourishment could be a trigger. Don't fall into the trap of choosing a food that they see as a real treat (otherwise you may find these tantrums happen more frequently) and avoid food with a high GI value such as biscuits, chocolate, cakes and sweets as these can aggravate their moods even more. It's best to offer something like a piece of fresh fruit or banana on a slice of wholemeal bread – even a packet of low-on-the-salt crisps isn't a bad option. A sandwich with a lean protein filling would be good too, as the protein helps to slow down the absorption of the carbohydrate in the bread and therefore enables their blood sugar level to be better controlled.

Eczema

Eczema is an inflammatory skin condition, which causes dry, itchy skin that can drive little ones wild enough to want to scratch and claw away at their bodies. This can make the skin break and bleed and can lead to secondary infections. Genes definitely play a part, but there are also environmental and lifestyle factors, as well as diet, that can have an impact on whether your child suffers from eczema. Eczema is far more common than we'd think and is not only a complex skin condition to treat, but as I've found over the last couple of years with Maya, can be distressing for us both.

There are so many triggers responsible for the skin flaring up and how eczema affects your child will vary greatly. It can range from the odd patch on their elbows and behind their knees to those who can be literally covered from top to toe, and need to have bandages on at night to soothe and protect bleeding limbs and to stop them scratching.

Read more on: ◆ Page 59
Children and babies over six months who suffer from eczema can eat the same foods as those recommended for pregnant and breastfeeding mums ◆. However, since most kids aren't that great at eating sardines, mackerel, herrings etc., if your child has eczema, I would also give your child an omega oil supplement containing 2g (2,000mg) of EPA and DHA. You can get some easy-to-swallow chewy capsules, but liquid forms

Organic food and farmers' markets

The recent debate over whether or not organic food is healthier for us than non-organic food has highlighted how complex an issue this is. One of the main problems is that it's very hard to compare an organic product with a non-organic one, while there are so many subjective factors such as how easy a food has been to source, how it tastes, how well it cooks, how it makes us feel, and what it has cost. In my opinion, there is little point in overstretching our budget for imported organic food if it doesn't cook well.

To qualify for organic status, farmers must adhere to strict regulations on artificial fertilisers and pesticides – pests and diseases are controlled using wildlife, and some farmers boost the nitrogen content of soils by planting clover. Livestock must be fed organic feed, have access to land for regular exercise (poultry must be free-range) and be kept in appropriate shelter. These conditions naturally reduce the risk of disease so drugs and wormers are only allowed in emergencies, which again many organic food eaters prefer. Lots of people who choose organic produce are sympathetic to this farming ethos.

Reports have shown that organic produce doesn't necessarily contain any more vitamins or minerals than non-organic food. The meat from an organic steak may not contain any more iron than a non-organic steak (so won't necessarily correct low iron levels in your body more effectively), but many people prefer to support smaller organic producers who are passionate about animal welfare. If the fact that the meat is organic makes you feel more comfortable eating it, then this simple fact will in the end benefit your iron status as you'll be eating more.

It angered me to see the report published in 2009 by the Food Standards Agency (FSA). Although this had promised a comprehensive review of scientific evidence, it included comments such as 'There is no evidence of additional health benefits from eating organic food.' I know the non-organic food lobby just loved to interpret this as evidence supporting the organic movement as a waste of time. But people need to look at the fine detail in the report and reach their own conclusions, taking what they did find into consideration: for instance, they found that in organic vegetables there was 53.7 per cent more beta-carotene as well as 38.4 per cent more flavonoids, 12.7 per cent proteins and 11.3 per cent zinc.

There has been a great deal of criticism over the methodology used in the FSA's research, and many people feel they didn't consider evidence from recent studies (although there was some concern over the scientific validity of some of the studies, which reported the nutrient levels of organic foods). However, we need to interpret the results in terms of the differences we value in own our lives.

The organic label, especially when we're talking about imported produce, which won't have the same high standards as ours, doesn't automatically mean that the food is healthy – processed meats and other organic foods can have high levels of saturated fats, salt and sugar. The legislation that surrounds how much of the food needs to contain organic ingredients in order to be able to call itself organic varies from product to product, so I always think it's best to check the labels of organic food in the same way as you would with non-organic produce. Products like organic cola and organic sweets made with just as high levels of refined sugar should be given just as wide a berth as non-organic. It's also worth bearing in mind that some producers haven't yet received their organic certification, but that doesn't mean their produce isn't of a high quality. On the other hand, not all free-range is organic – for example, free range chickens may be fed genetically modified feed. Again, it's always worth checking the label.

As to the argument that organic food tastes better than non-organic, this is a silly thing to say because it depends on each and every food. We all have the right to choose –

how I base my decision on whether to buy organic depends on the individual food and supplier, and I like to support some good organic food producers but I don't like to base my decision just on their organic label. For me, quality, price and whether the food has travelled from afar when I could have supported a good local supplier are all accounted for in my decision-making.

I am passionate about the good, clean, fair mission of the slow food movement, but do think that in recent years, the local farmers' market movement has slightly backfired. You get some good small producers selling great-quality foods at good prices but you can also find over-priced poor-quality food being sold in a trendy-looking market, which you would have been far better off buying from a supermarket. It angers me when people (especially those struggling with food budgets) get ripped off by market traders or are made to feel guilty for not feeding their family on locally produced market-bought produce. I shop in a combination of supermarkets, I use the Internet for getting to other smaller suppliers, and if I can, I go to a good farmers' market or support local suppliers for certain ingredients. I especially enjoy educating Maya about where food comes from and for her to see small producers at markets when we have the time.

are also available or you could crack open the capsules and mix them in with milk and juices if your child finds them unpalatable. You need to be patient, as it can take several weeks for the skin to calm down, and once their skin has improved they need to keep taking the supplement.

If your child can avoid the offending food allergen, their skin will dramatically improve. The most common are: milk (usually cow's milk, but could be sheep's or goat's), eggs, citrus fruits (usually oranges are the no-no), seeds, nuts (especially peanuts), shellfish, wheat, soya (yes, soya can be a problem too, in which case you might have to use rice, hemp or oat milk) and food additives (particularly the azo dyes and benzoate preservatives ◆). Non-food irritants that can aggravate eczema include: detergents, soap, shampoo, household chemicals, rough clothing, heat, scratching, hard water, house dust and house mites, moulds, pets and wool.

Read more on:
◆ *Page 111*

You need to weigh up the benefits – for just the odd patch of eczema behind the knee you might decide that other than trying to make your child's diet well-balanced, with some omega oil supplements thrown in for good measure, it's just not worth trying to get them to exclude foods. But for more serious eczema cases, changing their diet and avoiding the offending foods can be the only way to make life bearable. I would strongly recommend seeking professional advice from a paediatric dietitian if your child has severe eczema and you suspect that a food allergy may be aggravating it.

Probiotics and prebiotics

The word 'probiotic' means 'for life', but we're more used to hearing the term 'friendly bacteria'. We all have these bacteria living in our gut, some more than others, and their main purpose is to maintain a healthy digestive system. It's my view that if we can incorporate probiotics and prebiotics in our children's diets in an enjoyable and delicious way, we're at least nourishing them well for today and at best for a healthy future too. Stress, too much alcohol, too much junk food, IBS, cancer, diabetes and infections that necessitate taking antibiotics can all upset the balance of bacteria. Sometimes a week or so of not eating the foods we know to be nourishing can be enough to destabilise a child's gut flora enough to make them feel out of sorts. And of course if your child is under the weather their gut could do with a helping hand to rebalance the bacteria.

Most probiotics help digestion by breaking down tough fibres, enzymes and other proteins found in food. Probiotic bacteria are the resilient bacteria that can survive the stomach's acids and reach the intestine, where they benefit health-producing nutrients such as vitamin K and ferment organic acids, which are absorbed into the bloodstream for energy. They also play an important role in fending off more harmful disease-causing organisms known as pathogens.

Including live probiotic yoghurt in your child's daily diet is one thing, but it is possible to help your child's gut do much of the work for itself, without or as well as actively boosting the probiotic content of their diet. You can do this by incorporating prebiotic-rich foods, which can be seen as the 'grow-bag' for a healthy gut as they aren't digestible by the body's own enzymes, so they travel through the stomach unaffected. The two main prebiotics can be found in asparagus, bananas, barley, chicory, garlic, Jerusalem artichokes, leeks, milk, onions, tomatoes, wheat and yoghurt. Generally the fresher the vegetable the higher the amount of prebiotics, but we don't yet know how often we need to eat these foods, or how much – one onion may have a lot more prebiotics in it than another onion, for example, and there are no visual or labelling tell-tale signs.

If you have a child who is really struggling with their gut – constipation, diarrhoea or IBS – find either a combined prebiotic and probiotic or a specific prebiotic supplement. Some prebiotics are added to breakfast cereals, juices and yoghurts. Children may initially become a little windy when they start boosting their intake of prebiotic foods or powder, but this soon subsides.

There's no such thing as a miracle food

What's important to realise is that as with all foods, probiotics and prebiotics are not miracle workers. Just because a product (whether it is a tablet, a drink or a food) contains them doesn't mean it is all-round nutritious, as some are high in sugar. Since research has shown that probiotics can help treat diarrhoea (particularly in children) caused by antibiotics and tummy bugs, for me, this justifies trying to make my daughter's diet as rich in probiotics and prebiotics as possible. I have seen some kids who have taken probiotics following an episode of acute diarrhoea or constipation recover very quickly.

There is some research to show that taking probiotic and prebiotic supplements on a daily basis may also prevent food poisoning, improve symptoms of lactose intolerance, reduce susceptibility to skin problems such as eczema, help control IBS, strengthen the immune system and reduce cholesterol levels. I don't think we should all start dashing out and buying supplements because in order to be sure of maintaining a healthy dose of good bacteria in the gut, your child really needs to take probiotics indefinitely, which can be a hassle and expensive. So unless this is something you want to invest in every day, I'd suggest adopting an overall habit of including some probiotic natural yoghurt in their diet most days. Note that if your child is lactose-intolerant you need to check the label, as some supplements contain lactose.

Constipation

It's what every parent dreads – seeing your child in agony on the toilet is upsetting, especially when they're at such a sensitive stage in their lives. The whole issue of not being able to go to the toilet when they and you want them to can be a worry, and the last thing you want is for them to be afraid of going because it's so painful and then perhaps getting so blocked up that when they do go they have accidents or painful diarrhoea.

Sometimes when children are going through a tough time at school – with exams or bullying, for example – the body can exhibit this upset in their gut. They may complain of tummy ache, or have trouble going to or staying off the toilet. This is why when you're treating children for gut symptoms like this it's important to see if you can dig a little deeper as to how happy they are, and whether something needs to be sorted outside their diet (I've seen so many children with tummy problems whose parents have either started them on bizarre exclusion diets or sent them off for expensive, unnecessary and uncomfortable tests when really what's needed is some good old-fashioned listening and good eating). Getting back to proper eating habits should be the first priority, but alongside this you could also enlist the help of a probiotic supplement (and see if you can do more on the prebiotic side of their diet) to rebalance temporary upsets.

Food can be the cause and cure of children's gut problems as much as adults', so the more we can do to help them get over constipation, the better. If, having tried the tips on the following pages, your child still remains constipated, visit your doctor, who may prescribe a mild laxative. Don't abandon my nutritional advice, however, because the more you can help to relieve your child's constipation through food, the less you will rely on laxative drugs. Above all, remember to be relaxed about your child's eating and toilet habits. Uptight children are likely to develop bowel problems, so the more you can do to calm them down (and appear calm yourself), the fewer problems you'll all experience.

Read
more on:
◆ Pages
38–40

Pearled spelt
with broad
beans,
asparagus
& dill,
page 208

Make sure you boost their fluid intake. Dehydration can be one of the most common reasons why children get constipated so get them to drink plenty of plain water ◆. It doesn't matter whether the water is cold or room temperature, although sometimes room temperature water works better with a sore tummy. Plain water is the most hydrating, but if you need to make it a touch more interesting, mix it with a little fruit juice in the proportions of one third juice to at least two thirds water. Chamomile tea is very soothing for a constipated gut, so get them to try some either (safely) hot, or cooled. I like to add a little aloe vera to the water or juice – this natural plant extract can soothe a sore tummy and also loosen the stool to get things moving.

Lack of fibre is right up there with lack of water as a key reason why your child might be struggling to pass a stool. Fibre needs plenty of water to help it swell and stimulate the gut to move, so if you boost the fibre in their diet and not the water, you can make constipation ten times worse. Focus on boosting your child's fibre intake by choosing wholemeal bread, wholegrain cereals, oats, spelt, quinoa etc., plenty of fruits and vegetables (raw or cooked are both fine as fibre levels don't diminish with cooking), lentils, beans, seeds and nuts.

All fruits seem to have a particularly strong laxative effect. The most powerful ones are figs, dates, apricots, papayas, prunes, rhubarb and soft fruits such as plums and greengages, but whatever you can get your child to eat will help. You can buy small pots of prune-based fruit purée to use on cakes, pancakes, toast and ice cream. It's easy to make your own by simmering the dried fruit in a little orange juice until soft. Try not to see it as a medicinal thing – fruit purées are delicious. You could also give your child a small glass of prune juice every day, either on its own or mixed with freshly squeezed orange juice.

Check your child is not eating too much fast food. A diet too heavy in fast-fried ready-made food and not enough fresh vegetables and good home cooking is more likely to bung children up. This can explain why holidays can be a nightmare for their gut – their routine can be disrupted, especially if they're having to travel on planes for a long time and not only don't get much of an opportunity to roam around and get their gut muscles working but have to eat strange food at strange times. It's a hassle, but the more I travel with Maya, the more convinced I am that the answer is for me pack food for us to eat on the plane that we will both enjoy, and that we know will make us feel good at the end of the flight rather than the pre-packaged aeroplane food that is served.

Some children are allergic to, or intolerant of, wheat or dairy produce. If you suspect that your child has tummy troubles after eating a specific type of food, keep a food diary ◆ for a couple of weeks, making a

Read
more on:
◆ Page 11

Read

▲ Pages
170–171

Pan-roasted
Padrón
peppers,
page 228

record of when they go to the loo and any other symptoms such as headaches. Having analysed the food diary, if you think you can see a pattern, give your child less of the suspect food, and if this strategy has positive results, ask your doctor to refer you to a paediatric dietician for advice on how best to balance your child's diet. It may be something more serious such as coeliac disease ▲ so don't delay in speaking to your doctor if the symptoms don't improve.

Excess wind

Sometimes specific foods can trigger children to be more windy, as can too much spicy or fatty food. Keeping a note of what they eat and how their gut is can give you some pointers, but for use immediately if they've got it now, try some weak fennel tea. You can make your own or use a tea bag. Sometimes resting up, a warm bath or hot water bottle can help, but at other times getting them running around can get air moving in the right direction too.

A word of caution before you start taking specific foods out of your child's diet. I more often see good results with children when we look at a few simple things: Is your child sitting up straight when eating? Slouching makes it uncomfortable to swallow food and they end up swallowing a lot of air at the same time; try to get them to slow down with their eating – hard, I know, but fast eating means they generally put too much food in their mouth and then struggle to swallow it and end up overloading their tummy; try to discourage talking while they're eating, as this helps the digestive system work more efficiently and is less likely to lead to a windy, painful gut; make sure they're sticking to regular mealtimes and not eating too many snacks; look at the section on probiotics ◆, as sometimes wind is caused and aggravated by too many bad bacteria – especially if they've just finished a course of antibiotics or have had a cold; if you're tempted to start cutting out specific food groups since you suspect an intolerance, discuss it with your doctor, who can refer you to a dietitian for help; fennel tea is made with just a teaspoon of fennel seeds – simply infuse in boiling water for a couple of minutes, strain, and allow to cool to the right temperature.

Read
more on:
◆ Pages
104–105

Upset stomach

If sickness and diarrhoea lasts for more than 12 hours or if you're worried, call your doctor. If your child is being sick and passing loose or watery stools, keep them off food – much as they may cry out for something to eat, the last thing they need is anything inside more inside them, as it'll only come up or pass through again and cause stress to their gut when it's not in great shape. Try to get them to take regular sips of something liquid, as it's important to keep them as well hydrated as possible.

Tummy soothers

If your child has a tummy ache caused by a tummy bug or anxiety, first, I'd reach for ginger. You could try crystalline ginger, which you can buy in health food stores, to chew on, but this can be covered in sugar, so it's better to make fresh ginger tea. Grate some fresh ginger root, place in a small saucepan and cover with boiling water. Simmer for about eight to ten minutes then strain it and add some honey, or a little fresh lemon. If you pop it into their favourite mug to sip, the ginger can dissipate the tummy ache and nausea.

Honey

You may be a little curious as to why I said I didn't recommend crystalline ginger coated with sugar for kids, but on the other hand suggest adding honey to their tea. The reason for this is that although honey can be just as calorific as sugar, and when eaten on its own it can stick to teeth and cause tooth decay, when it's added to tea it loses its stickiness, so it shouldn't be as damaging for children's teeth. Honey also contains a few B vitamins, and when it's diluted in tea, your child won't get the same sugar hit as when chewing a sweet. If they have a sore throat caused by a virus, a teaspoon of room temperature honey, on its own, is the way to help them get over it.

Warning! Children under one year old shouldn't be given honey, as it may cause infant botulism.

Alternatively try peppermint, which has a strong antispasmodic effect and can take away tummy ache as well as wind: pop a few fresh mint leaves into a teapot and cover with boiling water. Again you can add some honey.

Finally Peter Rabbit's favourite, chamomile tea. You can either use a tea bag and let it infuse for three to five minutes, or use the dried flowers, which I like and which you can get from good health food shops. The dried flowers make a sweeter, honey-like tea – use just a pinch of the dried flowers and infuse in the boiling water for three to five minutes. Chamomile is also great for calming children down if they've come back from a party wired, or if they're over-tired and bouncing off the walls.

Attention Deficit Hyperactivity Disorder

It's pretty likely that there will be one or two children in your child's year group (boys are four times as likely to have the condition than girls) that, rightly or wrongly, have this label attached to them. If the classic symptoms of Attention Deficit Hyperactivity Disorder (ADHD) – insomnia, lack of concentration, moodiness and frequent destructive outbursts – sound familiar, then the first step is to talk to your doctor who can refer you to a paediatric team for expert assessment and advice. Although you may recognise traits and behaviour patterns which suggest to you that your child has ADHD, don't slip into the mistake of self-diagnosing, or equally accept a doctor's first diagnosis and drug prescription without having your child properly assessed by a specialist. It's far too easy to put the wrong label on a child, which will only result in incorrect treatment when perhaps psychological or nutritional therapy could be more effective.

It has to be said that some of the studies into the relationship that food plays in altering mood and behaviour throw up mixed results, but from my experience and those of many colleagues working in this area, changing the diet of children with ADHD can make a noticeable difference. Since the side-effects of dietary and behavioural change (apart from being hard work and needing lots of determination) are minimal, I urge all parents of children with ADHD or other behavioural issues to look at some key aspects of their diet. The first area to focus on is the general overall healthiness of the diet: small, frequent, healthy meals, lots of water, fresh fruits and vegetables and a high intake of essential fatty acids. It is also essential to strip out the baddies – too many of the high-GI foods and additives. With careful fine tuning of the diet, I have turned children with huge behavioural issues around, and the results can be literally life-changing.

Replacing high GI foods with wholegrains

Despite the fact that many parents swear that sugary foods turn their little ones wild, there is little scientific evidence to prove that they have a bad effect on behaviour. But my feeling is that since foods that are highly processed, overly sweet or have a high glycaemic index (GI) have little to offer nutritionally, it is worth trying a lower GI diet ◆. This may just help to reduce some of the symptoms, but will also benefit their health in so many other ways, such as making them less likely to be overweight and suffer from tooth decay. High-GI foods don't just include the obviously sweet foods like biscuits and cakes. In fact, as you will read throughout this book and see from many of the pudding and cake recipes, if you use wholegrain ingredients and use fruits as a base, you can make something scrumptious which shouldn't have as negative effect on their blood sugar levels as a refined, processed biscuit. It's also worth looking at starchy foods – white rice, white bread and boiled potatoes – to see if changing to wholegrain versions brings about any benefits as although the GI value in wholegrain versions of these food is still high, they offer a lot of other nutritional benefits and don't tend to have the same negative effects. I often warn my patients that changing their child's diet might make them more moody or lethargic to begin with, but this is just the stage of being weaned off the rapidly absorbed sugars. Within a few days they should start to find a more consistent energy level and hopefully you'll see some other positive mood and behavioural effects too.

Read more on:
◆ *Pages 146–148*

Smoked mackerel pâté, page 217

Additives

Manufacturers put some additives in our foods to stop them going off and to give good texture, but when it comes to children and additives, I try to keep well away from tartrazine (E102/FD&C yellow 5), quinoline yellow (E104/food yellow 13), sunset yellow (E110/FD&C yellow 5), carmoisine (azorubine) (E122/food red 3), ponceau 4R (E124/cochineal red A), allura red (allura red AC) (E129/food red 17) and sodium benzoate (E211). Both studies and my own experience have shown that kids who eat a diet free of these additives (in addition to looking at other areas of their diet and lifestyle) are much healthier, more evenly behaved and can concentrate better.

The salicylate issue

On rare occasions, children with ADHD have reacted to a group of naturally occurring chemicals known as salicylates. In such cases they should be referred to a paediatric dietitian. If you suspect a problem, you may want to try removing the salicylate-rich foods – apples, oranges, nectarines, tangerines, grapes, cherries, cranberries, peaches, apricots, plums, prunes, raisins, almonds, tomatoes, cucumbers, peppers – from your child's diet just for a few weeks to see if behaviour improves. It's a huge list of healthy foods, but if you notice your child craving and eating a lot of any item on the list, just try reducing the quantity to a more balanced amount into their overall diet. (I have to say that tomatoes are the only thing on the list that I've really experienced as a trigger.)

The goodies

Read more on:
◆ *Pages 17–18 & 95*
▲ *Page 11*

Wholemeal soda bread, page 237

Finally, but very importantly, one of the most exciting areas of research into the relationship between foods and behaviour focuses on getting children to eat more of the oily fish that are rich in omega-3 fatty acids ◆. The reason why oily fish come to the rescue is that they contain beneficial fatty acids, which positively influence the signals that are sent back and forth between the brain and parts of the body. EPA in particular has been shown in many studies to have the power to stabilise mood swings and generally improve mood, behaviour, concentration and learning abilities of children with ADHD. Vegetarian non-fish sources of omega-3 fatty acids aren't the long chain beneficial omega-3 fatty acids that have been shown to be most useful, so if your child is following a vegetarian diet, I would discuss giving them an omega-3 supplement with your doctor.

Sometimes kids with ADHD can have food intolerances, and avoiding these foods (most typically wheat or milk) can improve their behaviour. Ask to be referred to a paediatric dietitian for some professional support. I would stress how useful it is to keep a detailed diary of what your child eats ▲ for a good couple of weeks, as this can give you and any professionals from whom you seek advice a real idea of which foods could be aggravating the child's behaviour. Try to keep the diary as secret as you can, apart from asking them what they've eaten at friends' homes or at school, as they can quickly cotton on and start playing up which muddies the waters!

If this sounds daunting, remember that children with a short attention span will feel positively stimulated, interested and therefore better able to concentrate and behave well if they see their parents preparing different foods and then sitting down to eat as a family – this is just one example of how eating and behaviour modification are intertwined. If there is no way that your child will eat fruit or vegetables, give them a daily multivitamin and mineral supplement (one which lists the dietary reference values for the nutrients and is free of bad additives and E numbers) to ensure that their body receives some nutrients. It's particularly worth looking at zinc and iron supplements as low ferritin (iron store) levels have been associated with higher hyperactivity symptoms in children. This should make them feel better so that in turn their eating habits and behaviour improve.

The Middle Years

'What's happening to my body?' is a common thought as we hit our 50s and 60s. We may look in the mirror and see lines appearing, weight piling on and our body shape changing, all of which affects our confidence at a time when most of us need every ounce we can get. Typically both women and men find their middle starts expanding, and yet the bits we wish would preserve their voluptuousness, be this our breasts or bums, seem to lose their peachiness. These changes combined with not having as much get up and go as we used to, and often a lower libido and all that entails, means that the onset of middle age can cause considerable anxiety.

But enough of the doom and gloom – there are so many gorgeous, inspirational, men and women such as Richard Gere, George Clooney, Judi Dench and Isabella Rossellini, who I think are even more attractive now that they have grey hair and 'expression lines', as my darling calls them. In many ways, entering middle age can feel like you are being given a new lease of life. As our grown-up children move away and we prepare for retirement, we still have the energy and enthusiasm for life that keep us vibrant and beautiful. It can be incredible to see a patient turn from someone who feels that all the above changes are inevitable into a person who feels healthier and happier in every respect. I aim to guide you towards the foods that are spot on for your body now that it's entered the middle-aged stage.

Putting on weight

As we age, our body's energy requirement decreases, although there are times – if there are underlying health problems such as recovering from an operation – when the body needs extra. Many people mistakenly think that they are eating and exercising as they have always done, so can start to fill out. You may have seen headlines recently suggesting that according to some studies we should be restricting our calorie intake even more tightly in order to maintain an ideal body weight and body fat measurement. Although we do need to monitor our calorie intake I feel that (a) restricting it even further is not realistic, and therefore even the most determined would feel they were failing and (b) we shouldn't be wavering from the aim of enjoying nourishing, delicious foods. We face plenty of challenges in our work and family lives, and we certainly don't need to add food to our list of worries – food can give the greatest of pleasures at times when lots of things seem like hard work, and we need to retrain our bodies so that we follow healthy eating patterns.

Apple or pear and BMI

The body mass index (BMI) is used to determine whether a person is under or overweight. Although BMI gives us some idea of the health risks associated with being a certain weight for your height, it doesn't take into account a person's body fat content and is not as accurate if you're an athlete, pregnant or breastfeeding, very young or very old. Waist circumference and waist to hip ratios are now believed to be much more reliable measures of future health risk as it's the fat around our middle that poses most danger.

Most of us store body fat in one of two distinct ways – around our hips and thighs, or around our middle. Those who store fat around the middle are often known as having an 'apple shape' or 'beer belly', while those who store fat around the hips and thighs are known as having a 'pear shape'. The shape of your body is directly linked to your risk of poor health. Too much fat around the body increases our risk of developing heart disease, diabetes, stroke, breast and colon cancers, osteoarthritis and emotional problems such as low self-esteem and depression. Over the past few years, scientific research has demonstrated that being an apple shape puts a person's health at greater risk than being a pear.

Effect of hormones

Many of the changes that occur in our bodies in mid-life happen because our hormone balance begins to alter. The hormonal shifts that occur – for example, women's oestrogen levels and men's testosterone levels start to decrease – can mean that men lose muscle bulk, and may start putting on fat around the middle, while women may start noticing a spare tyre forming, or those dreaded bat wings under the arms. Muscle bulk, muscle strength and our skin's elasticity all change, which means we can pile on weight and start changing physically in ways we would prefer not to. Some body changes can be tackled by exercise alone, but mostly it's a combination of a good diet and exercise that gives us the greatest chance of success.

Exercise

Put simply, body fat gets deposited when we take in too many calories and don't burn up enough in our everyday life. We lead such sedentary lives now – I notice that even though I live in the countryside and spend a huge amount of time outside, gardening, walking and cycling Maya to school, there can be days when I find I've sat glued to the computer all day with only my hands doing any activity. We can be shocked at how little exercise and activity we do – in the same way as keeping a food diary ◆ , try keeping an activity diary for a couple of weeks and I bet you'll find that your diet is far too high in energy for the amount you expend.

Read
more on:
◆ Page 11

Quick Caesar
salad,
page 221

Exercise specialists usually recommend a combination of muscle development and aerobic fat-burning exercise, such as running, swimming, cycling and brisk walking, as not only do toning and muscle development exercises such as lifting light weights, yoga and pilates improve posture and body shape, but our metabolic rate can rise as our muscle mass increases. If we combine this with cardiovascular exercises, which are good fat-burners, slowly but surely our metabolic rate will climb and our body shape will start to head in the direction we want it to. People often worry about their weight, but in fact more health risks are linked to how much body fat we're carrying than what the scales say – this is certainly the case with heart disease, diabetes and certain cancers, specifically breast cancer. Okay, joints don't like having to work extra hard and energy levels might be lower if we're having to hoik a heavier body around, but if our weight is largely muscle and we're keeping our body fat levels within the ideal range it's highly likely our body's not going to run into half the health problems it would do if it was carrying too much fat.

Watch what you eat and drink

The easiest way to reduce our body fat level is to take a careful look at the concentrated sources of calories. The obvious one is fat, but it's not that simple – and indeed we need some good fats in our diet at this stage in life, to protect our bones, heart, etc. We need to look at the amount of refined sweet foods we're eating, and at our portion sizes of all foods – even if we're talking about a full-of-fibre wholemeal bread sandwich, if we eat too much of a good thing then our weight and our body fat will just stay too high.

The most calorie-dense foods are those rich in fat and sugar. On the sugar side, women going through hormonal changes may find they get raging sugar cravings that can get them into all sorts of trouble, as they're often pretty addictive and only satisfying for a few moments. We know how at different times in our menstrual cycle our body can crave sugar or chocolate, and the menopausal oestrogen shifts can sometimes bring these all back again even more strongly. You'll be particularly prone to sweet cravings if you're struggling with the emotional changes encountered at this stage of your life. In short I'd try avoiding all sweet foods other than fresh fruits. Go cold turkey on them all – you may well be shouting and looking at the biscuit and chocolate shelves like a crazed person for a few days, but if you keep walking, chanting a mantra or doing whatever helps to distract you, within 48 to 72 hours you'll be past the danger zone and won't need half as much will-power to resist. Alternatively, some people find sniffing a vanilla pod or essence good for breaking the sweet craving.

With our decreasing metabolic rate we sometimes don't need the same amount of food. Just step back and have a look – keep a food and emotions diary for couple of weeks and see if you're perhaps eating more than you need, not really through greed but because of the simple fact that you have always eaten this much. It could be that if you serve yourself less and eat it slowly, you could cut down your food intake enough to ensure your weight and body fat levels stay in check.

Read more on: ◆ Pages 40–41

Not only is alcohol incredibly high in calories but it increases our appetite, takes away our will-power to eat well, and has a tendency to make us pile on fat around the middle – the beer belly shape. Plus the health risks of drinking too much ◆, are serious and, particularly with women, underestimated and taken far too lightly. I'm not trying to come across as a killjoy, but it can be astonishing how cutting right down on the amount we drink, can have a very positive effect. It can help with decreasing body fat levels, increasing energy, improving sleep (helpful in combating hot flushes, anxiety, snoring or sleep apnoea), boosting our self-esteem and making us feel far younger in body and mind. I don't buy the excuse that there is so much social pressure in and out of the workplace to drink like a fish – there's too much known about the health risks of drinking too much, and work ethos has altered so that boozy lunches can easily be got around if there's a will to change.

Worrying weight loss

So often we associate hitting middle age with gaining too much weight, but this isn't always the case. Stress, depression, anxiety and unhappiness over the way our body is changing, along with the complexities of life around us (be this children leaving home, or parents becoming ill or dying), or being faced with a diagnosis ourselves, can all make the way we eat move in the opposite direction.

Weight loss without any obvious reason should always be checked with your doctor even if you're not feeling unwell in any other way. If you are suffering from depression, although it may seem a bonus to shift a few pounds at first, losing too much weight and not eating properly is only going to make it harder to come out the other side. Eating can be the last thing on your mind, and some drugs prescribed for depression can put you off your food, but try not to slip into poor eating habits ◆.

Read more on:
◆ *Pages 45–49*

If your weight is dropping too low and your appetite is off, often it's a case of forcing yourself to eat a little. Take up any invitations from friends and family to join them at mealtimes, and if they offer to stock up your fridge say yes! Not eating enough and low blood sugar levels will make you feel weak and reduce your appetite further, so it could be that small meals, almost snacks, will suit you better. But make sure they're nourishing – much better to have a slice of wholemeal bread with good-quality peanut butter and a small banana than a packet of biscuits.

Menopause

Many of us dread the word 'menopause', but I actually prefer it to the term 'change', which can make women feel that they shouldn't talk about the fact that their body is entering a new phase in their life. The menopause affects women in completely different ways, but the most common symptoms include hot flushes, sweating, insomnia, anxiety, impairment of memory and fatigue. Long-term consequences can include a decline in libido, osteoporosis, heart disease, even dementia, all linked to reduced oestrogen levels. The reason we now even hear people refer to the time leading up to the menopause as the peri-menopause is, I think, thankfully a result of women feeling more comfortable to discuss such a sensitive time in their lives.

The usual age to start going through the menopause is when we hit our late 40s or early 50s and it seems to have a more profound effect on women's bodies and the way they feel than men. Some women can sail through with only the odd hot flush, but others have a pretty miserable time: weight seems to pile on, emotions are all over the place and their body can start to look and feel old and tired. The physiological reason why the body starts changing in such a way is largely down to a drop in oestrogen production – but as with most hormones, once one of them starts to alter it can have a knock-on effect on other hormones. Some menopausal symptoms such as lack of libido and vaginal dryness can be exacerbated by low testosterone levels, so sometimes testosterone therapy can be given alongside the more common oestrogen and progesterone therapies. Indeed, having adequate testosterone helps us to maintain strong healthy bones and good levels of HDL cholesterol ♦. Women usually produce enough testosterone from their adrenal glands to ensure that these health benefits are covered, but it could be worth discussing with your gynaecologist whether a little testosterone top-up could ease menopausal misery. With the male menopause, testosterone therapy may help too.

*Read
more on:*
♦ *Page 29*
▲ *Page 124*
● *Page 149*

*Beans with
tomato,
coriander &
coconut milk,
page 206*

Female menopause

Two very important health issues come into the spotlight during these menopausal years. First, lower oestrogen levels can reduce our bone density by as much as two or three per cent during the five or so years after the menopause. This may not sound much in percentage terms, but it can be significant enough to put bones at a far greater risk of fracture as a result of developing osteoporosis ▲.

Second, it is the female hormones that provide a level of protection against heart disease and storage of fat around the waist. As women approach the menopause, their oestrogen level drops dramatically, so this protective effect disappears and puts the body at a similar risk to men. Women who are a pear shape may also find that their body changes into more of an apple, and weight starts to gather around the middle, increasing the risk of developing type 2 diabetes ●. Although it can appear to be less serious than type 1, studies are in fact now finding that this type of diabetes can cause blindness and kidney, heart and circulation problems when blood sugar levels aren't controlled. Since type 2 usually remains undiagnosed for longer, the likelihood is that the higher blood sugar levels will have a considerable amount of time to cause damage. Insulin-dependent type 1 diabetics tend to be regularly monitored by doctors and dietitians, and the issue of having to inject themselves tends to make sufferers take their health more on board, whereas type 2 diabetics can be a little more laissez-faire, leading to all sorts of problems. The good news is that we can make a dramatic difference to our likelihood of developing any of these conditions simply by watching the way we eat, treat our bodies and lead our lives.

Many women associate menopause and diet with soya and phytoestrogens – nature's oestrogen mimickers. There seems to be an absence of menopausal symptoms, in countries where diets are naturally rich in phytoestrogens, such as the Far East and Japan. This doesn't mean that one is responsible for the other or that Westerners metabolise and benefit from the phytoestrogenic foods in the same way. Genetics and environmental factors play a huge part in how our bodies react to specific foods, so as yet we can't say whether a diet rich in phytoestrogenic foods is beneficial to women going through the menopause or not. But it could be worth a try if you're really struggling, and indeed there are some positives about including some of these foods even if they don't have much of a positive effect on the symptoms you're trying to relieve: they're usually high in fibre and protein, low in saturated fats, and some women prefer the taste of soya milk to cow's milk. If you are vegetarian or vegan, soya-based foods like soya milk, soya yogurt, tofu, miso and tempeh can be an invaluable part of your daily routine. The sort of level some women seem to find beneficial is if they drink a couple of large glasses of soya milk each day. You might want to think about one of the calcium-enriched soya milks, because they can also be useful for helping to abate some of the bone effects of the menopause.

If soya isn't your thing, other sources of phytoestrogens include pulses (lentils, chickpeas, beans, etc.), beansprouts, peanuts, linseeds (flaxseeds) and yams (sweet potatoes). We don't know how much you need to eat to glean any benefits, which is frustrating and you also need to bear in mind that too many legumes such as lentils and beans may make you feel bloated. Fortunately this is usually just in the short term, as your body will adapt to these wondrous high-fibre foods so it's worth persevering. Research is far more definite about showing that when you're going through the menopause there is a lot to be said for focusing your diet around a variety of fruits and vegetables (I would try to have about eight portions a day, if you can). You should also aim to eat up to four 140g (5oz) portions of omega-3-rich foods a week ◆, as these can help ease

Read more on:
◆ Pages 17–18 & 95

Chicken & chickpea burgers, page 212

some of the hormone-induced symptoms such as hot flushes, breast tenderness and mood swings. Some women find cutting out caffeine helps the symptoms – studies don't back this up, but I'd still give it a try.

As you will have read at the beginning of this chapter, one of the most significant issues to watch when you enter this time in your life is not overdoing the calories, as not only is weight gain far more likely but your metabolism also changes. It's important when you're looking at beneficial foods such as oily fish that you cook them lightly and incorporate them into a light and healthy nourishing diet; piles of smoked salmon on a bagel smothered in cream cheese isn't going to help ease any hot flush – it'll just find its way right down to your midriff and stay there! If you can lose some pounds by eating little and lightly, the likelihood is that many menopausal symptoms will become less noticeable.

Male menopause

Although the way we eat and the amount of exercise we do can have a significant impact on how our bodies look and feel during middle age, hormonal changes that occur in a man's body can also be a major player. It's only been in the last few years that we've started talking about men's hormones, which may in part be down to the fact that there is now a male HRT, which doctors are becoming more familiar with. Men don't tend to suffer in silence or accept that low energy levels, a changing body shape, poor libido and sexual ability should be something just to put up with – and quite right too.

Hormone replacement therapy (HRT) is one option to consider if you have low testosterone levels, but first I just want to point you back to the beginning of this chapter to have a look through the nutritional watch points. Some of the symptoms you experience as a man when you hit middle age may not be down to a hormonal imbalance – it could be the way you're eating drinking and living. Getting fatter, feeling sluggish, low in mood, etc. need not be inevitable – I see many patients in their mid-50s or 60s who at first are resigned to the fact that it's middle age, yet within a few weeks they can turn the situation around.

Men can be brilliantly focused on getting their body into shape once they make the decision to do so – it's often a company medical showing up high LDL cholesterol or a friend being diagnosed with a heart problem or cancer, which can be the kick up the backside. Traditionally women still do a lot of the food shopping, cooking and organising, which can of course make it easier if they get on board with the lifestyle and food changes. It doesn't take long to experience the benefits – even a few days of eating well and exercising can get you off the starting block to feeling

Supplements and herbal remedies

Supplements and herbal remedies that are rich in phytoestrogens are marketed at combating menopausal symptoms. However, there is limited evidence as to whether a diet rich in phytoestrogens helps relieve symptoms such as hot flushes, so I'd urge you to discuss taking any herbs or supplements with your doctor or clinical dietitian. Some herbal remedies have been found to contain high levels of toxic metals and even steroids, and they can interfere with other medication, so it's not something to be dabbled with.

Some women swear by herbal remedies such as black cohosh, dong quai and ginseng for helping them through this rocky hormonal time, but others find they make no difference, which can be disappointing, especially when you're trying to stay away from the conventional hormonal replacement therapies.

younger and fitter, which when you're talking about libido, sexual function and energy levels can have a big impact.

Bone health

Bones continue to grow in density (with a good and continuous supply of calcium and vitamin D) until our late teens and early 20s. This is a particularly crucial stage in our bone health, so we should make a point of encouraging healthy eating and living at a time when many young people think that they can throw caution to the wind and not worry about it. If we build strong bones while we're young we reduce the risk of our bones becoming fragile when we're older. The effects of what we eat on our skeleton are powerful and wide-ranging. It's absolutely critical that we look at how we can optimise our bone health much earlier on in our lives in order to reduce the rate and impact of bone diseases such as osteoporosis. We tend to think of bones as being inanimate and something we can't really influence, but in fact our skeleton is very much a living part of us:

bone cells are busy throughout our lives manufacturing new bone, and this process, although most evident in childhood and the teenage years, continues to be vitally important throughout the rest of our lives.

Often we only start to think about our bones when we enter middle-age and doctors start suggesting bone scans or instigating discussions as to whether taking hormonal replacement therapy (HRT) is for you – bone protection is one of the benefits offered by HRT. Even if you don't have a high risk of osteoporosis, since this disease is largely preventable and at least the impact and severity of it can be reduced by eating and living well, this can be a good time to check up on how you're nourishing your bones.

Osteoporosis

Osteoporosis (also known as brittle bone disease) is a disease of the bone which is characterised by a low bone mass and deterioration in the structure of the bone which ultimately causes the bones to become fragile and more likely to fracture. Not only can osteoporosis cause a great deal of pain and discomfort, especially when fractures happen, but also the costs of looking after people who suffer osteoporotic fractures (most commonly the hips, wrists and spine) are enormous. Yet it is largely preventable – how we eat, live and exercise has an enormous impact on how healthy our bones are. Therefore, by looking at nutritional factors that influence how dense and how fragile our bones are, this gives us a real way forward in trying to reduce the risk of suffering from osteoporosis.

We need to pay particular attention to our bone health after the age of 50 because, particularly in women when we reach the menopause, our bone density rapidly decreases – we lose an average of about 2–3 per cent over the next five to ten years, the loss being at its greatest in the early post-menopausal years ◆. There is a strong genetic link that can place us more at risk of developing osteoporosis, while smokers, people who aren't physically active (couch potatoes as they're so often referred to), people who have a lower than ideal body weight or eating disorder, people with bowel and digestive or kidney problems, or have to take regular medication such as corticosteroids or anti-convulsants are also more at risk than others.

Read more on:
◆ Pages 119–122
▲ Page 20

Roast mackerel ith potatoes & thyme, page 215

Calcium for healthy bones

Dairy produce has always been highlighted as the best source of calcium, but some people can't take it, either because they have a lactose intolerance or are allergic to cow's milk protein, while others just don't like eating dairy foods. Luckily, there are a few other sources to tuck into, which lately we've found to be pretty good at providing the body with easily-absorbed calcium ▲.

One frequent dilemma women can struggle with is balancing the need to eat enough calcium-rich foods to keep up their bone density without having too much high-saturated dairy food, which can increase levels of LDL cholesterol. Lower-fat dairy foods can be helpful as they not only contain less saturated fat and therefore don't increase your production of LDL cholesterol ◆ but in fact, low-fat milks contain slightly more calcium than the full-fat versions.

Read more on:
◆ *Page 29*
▲ *Page 20*
● *Pages 20–21*

Cauliflower cheese, page 209

I'm generally not a lover of low-fat products, as I think the taste falls down and some heavily-processed low-fat foods can be filled with sugar to make up for the missing taste bud-satisfying fat. To get the right balance, choose a dairy food that tastes good, such as a natural yoghurt or fromage frais. The fat content of yoghurt seems to vary a lot – from the runny no-fat variety, which I find disappointing, to the Greek-style yoghurts which can be up to 12 per cent fat. Although they're higher in fat I tend to go for the latter, as they're more satisfying, so you don't feel the need to eat so much. The best solution would be to find something in the middle that you enjoy.

Cheeses that are lower in fat include Gouda, Emmental, Parmesan, fromage frais, fresh feta, ricotta and cottage cheese. The fat content of goat's and sheep's milks varies, but it's harder to source lower-fat versions of these less popular dairy milks. The non-dairy sources of calcium ▲ are all good things to include in your diet, but I don't think their contribution is good enough to meet your calcium requirement at this stage in your life, especially if you have low bone density or have been diagnosed with osteoporosis.

Vitamins and minerals

Our bones need magnesium ● and although, I'm not fond of counting our food in milligrams of this or micrograms of that, the recommended daily intake for magnesium is 270mg for women and 300mg for men, which equates to 66g (½ cup) of Brazil nuts or 100g (¾ cup) of pine nuts. This is an awful lot to incorporate into your diet, so it may be where a combined calcium, magnesium and vitamin D supplement could work for someone who has low bone density, other strong risk factors, or for anyone who doesn't eat much dairy.

Vitamins K and D are also essential for bone health. If you're over 65 and can't absorb enough vitamin D from the sun, you need to take 10mcg (400 IU). If you suspect that your vitamin D status may be low or you have low bone density, discuss the issue of taking a supplement before you reach this age with your doctor.

Caring for our bones

We all need some fat in our diet to support the absorption of essential vitamins and some minerals, but we also need to have enough fat on our bodies to ensure that the hormonal environment is conducive to helping to protect our bones. A small amount of fat on your body helps to cushion the effect of a fall, making a fracture less likely, but too much fat hinders the way we can move. Falling when we're overweight can place an enormous load on our bones and therefore increase the risk of a fracture, and we can be less successful at manoeuvring our body into a safer falling position. It helps to ensure that your body weight is within the ideal range and that the type of fat you choose is as healthy as possible ◆. Although studies don't yet tell us why, it's thought that the fatty acids within oily fish and the vegetable-based oils help to support good bone health.

Read more on:
◆ Pages 17–18
▲ Page 44

It's another place where the studies don't give us strong evidence either way, but we do know that high salt intakes have been associated with an increase in the amount of calcium we lose in our urine. If we bear in mind that too much salt also has a negative effect on our heart health, I think it's a good opportunity to see how you can keep your intake down ▲.

Bones don't like too much alcohol. Chronic alcohol abuse tends to damage the cells that manufacture new bone and also interfere with the way our livers behave, which can have a profound impact on the metabolism of key nutrients such as calcium and vitamin D.

Finally, too much caffeine isn't good either, as it can interfere with the amount of calcium we absorb, so enjoy a small amount of good-quality caffeine-rich food or change to something caffeine-free. Some people I see with diagnosed low bone density or osteoporosis, or who really want to maximise the amount of calcium their body can absorb, prefer to give up caffeine altogether. But equally, studies don't show that a couple of caffeine drinks a day will do any harm to your bones.

Weight bearing exercise

Smoking and being inactive can severely harm your bones, and it's particularly important on the exercise side to include some load-bearing exercise – brisk walking, jogging, running, aerobics, boxing – something in which your body is placing a downward load on your bones. Yoga and Pilates can help you to move more easily and protect yourself from falling badly so do have a role to play in reducing the risk of fracture. However, when it comes to their efficacy at stimulating the bone cells to manufacture new healthy bone, they are not as efficient as load-bearing exercise. I would suggest a combination of different types of exercise, some load-bearing and some to increase your flexibility.

Tahini

Tahini is a thick paste made out of sesame seeds that's commonly used to make Middle Eastern dishes such as hummus, babaganoush (roasted aubergine dip) and halvah (a very sweet dessert). I prefer to go for the Greek or Lebanese brands rather than those in health food shops and supermarkets, which use unhulled sesame seeds and tend to be overpowering and heavy. It conveniently keeps for weeks in the fridge if sealed, but will go rancid if left opened in a warm cupboard. It's a source of calcium, but also of some protein, B vitamins, iron and essential fatty acids. However, it's laden with sesame oil, which, although mainly the healthier type of unsaturated fat, is hefty in calories, so don't overdo it.

I like to make it into a sauce by taking 150ml (⅔ cup) of tahini paste along with the same amount of water, 80ml (⅓ cup) lemon juice, two peeled cloves of garlic and a pinch of salt, and mixing them all together in a blender until smooth and creamy. Then I add about 25g (1 cup) of finely chopped flat-leafed parsley and mix well. I use this sauce on vegetables or as a sort of pesto-style dressing for salads or on cooked roast meats like chicken.

Water and waterworks

Ideally, you should continue to drink a couple of litres (quarts) of water every day. However, you may find that as your bladder, kidneys and pelvic floor muscles (for men the prostate gland) age, your ability to do anything other than visit every public convenience in the country is compromised! Women can strengthen their pelvic floor muscles by doing regular exercises, which should help you to cope with drinking a lot of water. Night-time waking and needing to go to the bathroom can be troublesome even if you don't drink that much, so you may well find that if you suddenly up your water intake in the hope of having all the health benefits of being well hydrated, going to the toilet all the time becomes a real pain. I would suggest that you take a few weeks to increase your water intake gradually – concentrating the increase during the day, as opposed to downing a lot with your evening meal. This gives the kidneys time to acclimatise to the increase in water intake, so that eventually you should be able to drink close to the ideal two and a half litres (10 cups) a day without too much disruption to sleep ◆ .

Read more on:
◆ *Pages 38–40*

Reducing our health risks

Avoiding the diseases we dread, such as cancer, heart disease, dementia and diabetes, can sometimes seem an overwhelming and impossible task. However, there are specific nutrients and foods that are particularly good for helping us do this if other aspects of our lifestyle, and health or strong genetic factors, make us vulnerable. But the pillar principles – eating at least five portions of fruits and vegetables a day and small amounts of good fats etc. – are essential before we begin to look at other areas of our diet.

Healthy brain

The reason I wanted to mention dementia in this chapter is simply because so many aspects of it – the diagnosis, treatment and day-to-day living with the disease – should be addressed as early as possible. Some of the drug treatments can have quite profound effects on slowing down the disease, and when it comes to nutrition, as with so many scenarios in our lives, the better nourished we are, the less likely it is that other complications will arise and the healthier, stronger and happier we'll feel. I cover it in much more detail in the last chapter ◆ but I think we can do a huge amount in our 50s and 60s to prepare our bodies for old age. Having a healthy body not only reduces the risk of developing certain diseases, but the symptoms are more manageable and we recover more quickly.

Read more on:
◆ *Pages 189 & 195–197*
▲ *Page 44*

Watch your salt intake

Ensure that the amount of salt you eat is reasonable ▲, as the risk of both high blood pressure and other heart-related problems increases with age. Too much salt can cause high blood pressure, and also aggravates bone loss and fluid retention, which some women find is a side-effect of taking HRT. Our feet can swell more than they used to when we were younger, which can be a sign of heart or other health problems, so if it's persistent check in with your doctor.

Bother with bowels

You may find that as your hormone levels alter your bowel habits also start to change – typically you may have been as regular as clockwork until you hit this middle-aged zone. The majority of bowel problems can be sorted by tweaking your diet, but it's worth finding out about constipation and irritable bowel syndrome (IBS)◆.

Read more on:
◆ *Pages 171–172*

Bowel cancer affects thousands of people and claims many lives every year, yet is completely curable if caught early and treated quickly. If you're at all worried by your change in bowel habit or have bleeding, abdominal pain or have lost a lot of weight and feel exhausted, see your doctor – the words 'bowel' and 'cancer' aren't often talked about, and it can lead to some people going around with symptoms which should be investigated but aren't. Don't just think it's IBS and something you have to put up with.

Preventing cancer

Developing cancer continues to be one of the most common worries we harbour about our health, and the anxiety increases as we get older – not just because cancer risk increases with age, but because it's pretty likely that even if we don't suffer from cancer ourselves, we know someone who has it now or has had it in the past. In fact it's estimated that more than one in three of us will develop some form of cancer at some point in our lives, so its impact continues to be significant.

The incidence of the different cancers varies hugely, but the four most common cancers (breast, lung, bowel and prostate) make up over half of all cases. A lot is talked about breast cancer, and it continues to be one of the most common types, but I also want to highlight the enormous number of people who are diagnosed with bowel cancer every day, with men and women being fairly equally affected. However, despite numerous campaigns and headlines being placed across the news broadsheets, we still seem to have an inordinate problem in talking about bowels. When a woman finds a lump in her breast she is highly likely to get straight on to seeing her doctor, but the problem with bowel cancer is that we often don't feel a lump. Since our gut is so often changeable, from times when we're completely fine to when constipation causes us grief or food seems to go straight through us, to go and talk to a doctor about our bowels just doesn't come easily to many of us. Often, therefore, the disease goes undiagnosed for a long time, and I fear that more and more people will go on without noticing the symptoms ▲ or addressing the problem. So it's up to us to become more familiar with our bodies and to be persistent with seeking the right specialist care if we have any worries over our bowels.

A massive two-thirds of bowel cancer cases could be prevented by eating, drinking and living well, but this is not to say that if you are diagnosed with bowel cancer or any other type you should think it's all

Read more on: ▲ Pages 131

Fruity beetroot cake, page 254

down to the way you've been living your life. Cancer is a complex disease, and there are many, many factors that influence whether or not you get it. Smoking should perhaps be put in a box of its own, since we all know that being a smoker takes your risk of developing cancer right up. To throw a figure around, smoking 20 cigarettes a day increases your risk of developing lung cancer by a massive 2,000–4,000 per cent, but our genes, where we live and the type of work environment we're exposed to, also play a large part.

We do know that by eating a certain way we can significantly reduce our risk of some types of cancer. The strongest links between cancer risk and what we put into our mouths is with bowel cancer, but it also applies to other parts of our digestive system, from the mouth, throat and stomach to the most common type of cancer, breast cancer.

The 'cancer-preventing' storecupboard

Surprise, surprise, fruits and vegetables are at the top of the list! As with all areas of science, studies differ in how effective certain foods are in preventing cancer. We do know, however, that eating healthily – and particularly fruit and vegetables – help to reduce the risk of certain cancers, including those of the mouth, throat, stomach and lung. We don't know exactly why, but they house a plentiful supply of nutrients and what we call bioactive substances (these are in a way 'super nutrients' found in plants which have a very positive effect on our health). It's the combination of all these nutrients that gives these foods specific antioxidant properties, which help reduce the impact of free radicals and cigarette smoke, which can trigger abnormal behaviour within cells and lead to cancer developing.

Fibre seems to be a key component in reducing the risk of certain cancers, particularly bowel cancer, because of its stool-bulking effect. Producing an easy-to-pass stool decreases the amount of time that waste products and toxins, which can cause some cell changes, spend in the bowel. Fibre also undergoes useful fermentation (brought about by the presence of bacteria) in the bowel, and in doing so produces what we call short-chain fatty acids, including one type called butyrate. This may all begin to sound a little complicated, but the long and the short of it is that fermentation protects the cells from changing in the wrong way – so fibre on all fronts should be something we treasure in our diet ◆. So we should be eating a plentiful supply of fruits and vegetables – this is where the five-a-day mantra comes from ▲, as we know this is the sort of level we should be getting through.

Read more on:
◆ Pages 30–32
▲ Page 16

You will see many adverts for vitamins and minerals which imply that they hold the answer to staving off diseases such as cancer. I can

Detecting bowel cancer

If you notice any of the following changes and they last longer than four to six weeks you should report them to your doctor. These symptoms are unlikely to be caused by cancer, but it's better to play safe.

- Bleeding from the bottom without any obvious reason.
- A persistent change in bowel habit to looser or more frequent bowel motions.
- Tummy pain, especially if severe.
- A lump in your tummy.

understand that it may appear easier and more scientific to take a pill, but not only do we know that the body finds it easier to absorb some nutrients when they're eaten as part of a normal diet, but research shows an increased risk of some cancers in people taking specific antioxidant supplements in large doses. This is not to say that taking a general standard multivitamin or mineral is going to harm you, but neither is it going to benefit you as much as eating a diet rich in fruits and vegetables.

Does meat cause cancer?

The two words 'cancer' and 'meat' seem to have appeared together in many health headlines, but it's a bit more of a complex relationship than it can initially appear. While studies have suggested that a high consumption of red or processed meat – bacon, ham – is linked with an increase in the risk of colorectal (or bowel) cancer, the evidence is a lot stronger for a link between a diet heavy in processed meats than if we ate some really good-quality lean steak a couple of times a week. There is a huge difference between a diet of processed poor-quality meat (whoever wants to eat that stuff anyway?) and the quality kind, but good-quality lean red meat seems to have been thrown into the same pot as the poor-quality, fatty stuff. The reality of being able to eat good-quality meat alongside a diet rich in fruits, vegetables and wholegrains is shown in studies to be completely fine, and indeed lean red meat provides us with some easily absorbed iron and omega-3 fatty acids. Okay, we can get these omegas from oily fish, but there is a lot to be said for including some good-quality lean meat in your diet if you would like to.

There is a wide spectrum of processed meats, from the kind that is not so great for us to eat, to the kind that is not so bad for us as long as we don't eat too much of it. Overall, studies suggest that eating about 50g (2oz) of processed meat a day (around two slices of ham or a slice of bacon) may increase the risk of bowel cancer by around 20 per cent, but they don't really distinguish whether they're talking about a piece of cheap salami or a slice of well-reared pancetta. So it leaves us a little in the dark – although for me this just makes a stronger case for choosing our meat well and eating a smaller amount of good quality. To put the role some meats can play into perspective, studies suggest that by smoking 20 cigarettes a day our lung cancer risk is 100–200 times greater than the effect of eating more than the recommended amount of processed meat!

In studies too (I don't want this chapter to be too study-heavy, but for me it shows how complex a subject area the whole relationship between cancer and what we eat is), we use the term 'red meat' to include pork, lamb, beef and processed meat. Scientists advise us to limit our consumption of processed meat and to keep our consumption of red meat to 500g (18oz) a week or less, which gives us real scope for enjoying delicious meat-based meals. Bear in mind that a bolognese sauce made with 500g of lean, good-quality beef mince should serve six hungry adults.

Salt and cancer

Health campaigns highlight the relationship between eating too much salt and ill-health, such as aggravating blood pressure and the loss of calcium from our bones, and attention is also drawn to the role it can play in increasing our risk of developing cancer. As you'll read in numerous sections of this book ◆, I am not an anti-salt queen – for me there is little point in having food which is bland, and sometimes we just need a pinch of salt to bring out great flavours.

Read more on: ◆ Page 44

When it comes to salt's relationship with cancer, studies are in their infancy, but we've found that the stomach can be more likely to fall prey to cancer if you have a high-salt diet. Smoked foods can be some of the worst culprits – this includes, unfortunately, delicacies such as smoked fish – herring, mackerel and salmon – and rashers of bacon and ham, so watch your consumption of these. There isn't any need to avoid them completely, just be mindful that you should try not to have too much, and should serve them with something fresh like a big, leafy salad packed with lots of raw vegetables.

Give your body a dose of wholegrain goodness as well – I think healthy, nutritious eating is all about knowing that if you have something, say, salty, fatty or sugary, you partner it with a food that is right up there in its almost-holiness. So a few slices of smoked salmon on warm wholegrain bread, served with a big watercress, raw spinach and tomato salad, is far better for you than if you have the same smoked salmon with white bread, a poor quality margarine, and a bag of crisps. This is why I think it's not always altogether helpful to look at labels on processed foods and feel that you have to go for the lower salt version, as sometimes it's bland. I'd rather have a smaller amount of a higher-salt food and make sure that the rest of my diet evens it out.

Cancer and weight

Not so talked about is the relationship that exists between carrying too much weight and cancer, but it's there, and significantly so when we look at specific cancers such as oesophagal, bowel, pancreatic, endometrial (the lining of the womb), kidney, gallbladder and breast (in post-menopausal women). To put a context on the risk, men are a staggering 50 per cent more likely to develop bowel cancer if their weight rises and puts them into the obese zone, while the figure for women is 25 per cent.

As to how much exercise we need to do, while the recommendation is for at least half an hour five times a week, I sometimes think this sort of statement makes us feel as if it's not worth doing any less than this, which just isn't the case. Something is always better than nothing, even if it's cycling to work, or getting off the bus a few stops early and walking. It can be shocking to realise how inactive a life we lead as we try to cram everything in, so think of exercise as a good thing in order to see if you can just make your everyday life less sedate and your cancer risk factor will go down.

The drink factor

I think we've been placing a little too much belief in the powers of the antioxidants which exist within the bottle – both the supplement tablets on the health food shelf and the alcohol we drink. Seldom a week passes without a headline discussing the beneficial antioxidant properties of beer or red wine, the oldest antioxidant shouter. We now know that it's only in the laboratory setting that red wine's antioxidants offer us any real benefits, and I suspect that the other types of alcoholic antioxidants won't fare any better.

Not only is it not good to see alcohol as a cancer preventer, but studies find a convincing relationship between drinking too much alcohol and the development of mouth, throat, oesophagus, liver and bowel cancers. Alcohol is a key factor in increasing the risk of breast cancer in women, and unfortunately we seem to be seeing some pretty worrying drinking habits.

Headlines and news items highlight binge drinking teenagers getting into all sorts of trouble, but I'm far more concerned about women in their middle age, as this is a far more private style of drinking, one that seems to have become part of our society. Women can buy wine very easily and cheaply, and it can be so easy to get into the habit of opening a bottle in the early evening or to share a bottle or two when eating out. The strains that life places us under when we hit middle age – elderly parents, children leaving home, a pressurised workplace – can cause the drinking habits of many a woman at this stage in her life to place her at risk of a lot of health issues, and cancer is right up there with them. I say this because I don't think we shout loudly enough about the dangers of drinking, especially for women, and yet ironically some women set their minds at looking to super-nutrients in health food shops but don't think about their alcohol intake ◆.

Read more on:
◆ *Pages 40–41*

Milk and cancer

There has been a lot of confusing information in the newspapers recently about dairy products and cancer, and in my opinion it's a case of watching and waiting for more clear research to come to light. Recent research shows that a higher intake of calcium (found in dairy products) can protect against bowel cancer, but some early research also suggests that there could be a link between dairy intake and the risk of developing prostate and ovarian cancers. For breast cancer the evidence is conflicting. A link between breast cancer and dairy products has been suggested, possibly because of the saturated fats they contain, or contaminants that could be present, but there is no clear evidence to support this. Another theory is that dairy products might help protect against breast cancer, but again, this needs to be backed up by firm evidence.

A large study called European Prospective Investigation of Cancer (EPIC) is currently looking at the relationship between diet, lifestyle and cancer. It will produce reports on diet and lifestyle and a variety of cancers over the next ten to 20 years, starting with bowel cancer and breast cancer. For the time being I believe that we should continue to include some dairy foods in our diet, as they're such a good supplier of calcium. If we incorporate all the other key food groups like fruits, vegetables and wholegrains, we'll get a good spectrum of nutrients which should balance each other out – remember, the healthiest diet is one that includes variety right across the food groups◆.

Read more on:
◆ *Page 14*
▲ *Page 123*

Soya and other phytoestrogens

Phytoestrogens are chemicals found in plant foods (phyto means 'plant'). They have a similar structure to the female sex hormone oestrogen and have been found to influence the effects of the menopause ▲. There are different types of phytoestrogens – some are found in soya bean products (isoflavones), whereas others are found in the fibre of wholegrains, fruit, vegetables and flax seed (lignans).

The main type of phytoestrogens in the western diet are lignans – so we're talking about foods like wholemeal bread, fruits and vegetables as opposed to soya bean products, which most of us don't eat that much of. However, these soya isoflavone types of foods seem to be the ones that are attracting the most research, as in certain parts of the world the diet is very heavily soya-based and the results of rates and types of cancers require some in-depth exploration. Whether soya is good or bad seems to be one of the hottest-contested and debated topics surrounding cancer, so I feel it requires a bit of space here.

A joint study was reported in July 2002 by Cancer Research UK, the National Cancer Institute of the USA and the National University of Singapore, which found that women with a soya-rich diet had breast tissue that was less dense than that of women with a low-soya diet. Higher density breast tissue has been linked to a higher risk of breast cancer, so this is the first study to directly link eating soya with an effect on breast tissue. Asian women, who eat the highest amount of soya foods, were found to have a lower risk of breast cancer. However, it's not clear whether genetic make-up (which influences the way that the body metabolises food) and environmental factors interact with the soya and therefore produce different effects in the body. What we can say is that in other parts of the world, most women do not eat enough soya to reduce their risk of breast cancer.

How to deal with cancer

Food has the power to nourish, so understanding what your body needs can be a key way to enhance the effects of conventional cancer treatment. Focusing on your diet if you have been diagnosed with cancer can be therapeutic in so many ways. It can not only provide key nutrients that can help your body fight the cell changes that cancer triggers, but also being able to take control of something yourself can have a positive effect on how you feel. The challenges you face when you're diagnosed with cancer vary considerably, from having to undergo surgery to enduring chemical or radioactive therapies, and it would be hard to cover them all in this chapter. But I want to take you through a few key ideas I've developed during the time I've been treating people with cancer, in the hope that they inspire you to see food, nutrition and nourishment as something positive and empowering on which to draw.

Some oncologists and cancer care surgeons and physicians don't consider diet to have any positive role to play in cancer treatment, which saddens me, because it's such a shame that some doctors put people off from exploring how food can be a great healer in its holistic sense. Although it's unlikely that eating a specific food will cause any significant change, in its truest medical sense, what you eat can not only support your immune system but can help a great deal with many of the unpleasant side-effects of the treatment, from a sore mouth to feeling sick, puffy, bloated and exhausted. Understanding everything there is to know about food and nutrients can help to relieve suffering and make the difficult relationship between cancer, eating and illness just a little easier. Doctors have hit out at pseudo-nutritionists who tell patients they can fight cancer without the need for medical intervention, and despite us having some supportive findings that the way we eat can have a positive effect on our immune systems, pseudo-nutritionists shouldn't lay claim to this. Of course there are instances when people have turned their back on conventional medicine and eaten their way to recovery by following diets that are bizarre and pure as they see it. We can't explain why these things happen, but turning their back on conventional treatment can be a worrying scenario for many cancer care surgeons and physicians, who would much prefer their patients to see nutritional intervention as a complementary therapy rather than an alternative. And this is exactly where I stand.

Tandoori chicken, page 213

Some doctors are also concerned when patients start to blame their cancer on a food they've eaten, or worry when their appetites change. Because the patients have heard from somewhere that white bread and pasta is bad when you have cancer, they can start worrying unnecessarily if they can't stomach wholegrains or any raw fruit or vegetables. Just as we know that nutrition has a positive role to play in helping to get our bodies in the right space to fight cancer, we also know that worry and angst don't do much to help. It doesn't matter if you have some days when you just fancy or can only stomach plain pasta or rice, or can just about manage to eat a biscuit – no food is going to harm you. As to the mad notion that's bandied about saying that sugar feeds cancer cells, so you should avoid all forms of sugar (fruit included), this is utter nonsense! All cells need sugar for energy – it's a simple biochemical reaction that supports life in every cell – so to say that you should stop all sources and provision of sugar to your cells, be these cancer or non-cancerous, is as crazy as saying that because all cells require oxygen we should stop breathing to prevent abnormal cell activity. So, let's move on to how best to eat when you're undergoing chemo and biological therapies (including vaccines and monoclonal antibodies), hormone therapies and other cancer drugs.

It has to be said that not all cancer treatments cause side-effects such as sickness and heart burn; how you feel could be down to the cancer itself, or to other drugs you're taking, such as painkillers or antibiotics. It's also important not to assume that sickness is definitely going to happen, or that if it does you should suffer in silence. Managing side-effects of drugs and symptoms is a key part of your oncology team's role, so don't be afraid to keep asking for their advice. After saying all this, feeling sick, even if you're not actually sick, is a pretty common side-effect of many cancer treatments (and of course anxiety can put us off our food too), so the more you can do to try to reduce your anxiety levels the more you may find that the intensity of the nausea waves lessens.

A note on cancer treatment

If you are undergoing treatment for cancer, there may be times when your immune system is particularly challenged – the cancer itself can also reduce your ability to fight what you would normally be able to ward off. So you need to be particularly careful about food hygiene, and also about avoiding the foods that carry a higher risk, such as raw eggs, and unpasteurised dairy products like milk and cheese.

Depending on how compromised your immune system is (your medical team can keep you up to date on your blood results), you may just need to eat cooked fruits and vegetables rather than raw, for the time being. The heat and the time the food is cooked for helps to reduce the bacterial content of food, so it's ideal to just eat freshly prepared cooked foods: a soup made from chicken broth, with some strips of soft chicken breast and noodles can have so much more nourishment in it and be tolerated far better than a chicken nugget cooked by a fast-food outlet. An oaty fruit crumble can give your body some much-needed fibre antioxidants, such as beta-carotene, if you make it with plums and blackberries, while a bowl of fruit compote with some thick Greek-style yoghurt can be refreshing, delicious and full of safe-to-eat goodness.

Nausea

Read more on: ◆ Pages 67 & 69

When experienced as a side-effect of cancer treatments, feeling sick is completely different, but I suggest that you begin by reading about morning sickness during pregnancy ◆, as so many of the tips I give there can help if you feel queasy. Because your immune system is being

The case against meat

The production of meat, especially beef, has a profound effect on global warming, not only because it requires astronomical volumes of water to produce but also because gases given off by cattle significantly contribute towards the greenhouse effect. It is always a good idea to consider the meat source and production process, although in reality, this should apply to everything we eat, not just meat.

Globalisation plays a huge role in the meat debate. Supermarkets search far and wide for cheap suppliers, often ignoring the increase in food transportation-related pollution. For example, living in Britain you would ideally choose British over New Zealand lamb and British over Danish bacon, but you may also consider whether or not the produce is organic – it's up to you to decide where your priorities lie. Foreign produce is not to be rejected per se – it is sometimes the only option, but try to weigh up the distance it has travelled over your necessity or desire to buy it. The best option is to buy local produce as often as possible, and that really does mean local, as much of the national goods supplied are sent to various different distribution centres all over the country. Don't forget that you're also more likely to receive fresher food if you buy it from local sources.

Since 1950, worldwide production of meat has increased fivefold, yet this is unsustainable – water and soil resources are being polluted and rapidly depleted. Meat is often intensively reared to cut costs, paying no attention to animal welfare. Apart from the question of animal rights, intensively-reared livestock is often kept in unhygienic and unnatural habitats, leaving livestock in a poor condition and reducing the quality of the meat. Crops used for animal feed are routinely grown using huge amounts of fertilisers and pesticides, and the animals themselves are often fed antibiotics to prevent diseases. These can enter the food chain and cause all sorts of problems in humans. In the last few decades, there have been several serious health scares involving meat. Bovine spongiform encephalopathy (BSE), E. coli and salmonella all pose threats to us, particularly to the young and the elderly. Regulations have been put in place to avoid contaminated meat, but the risk cannot be completely removed. If we take action to avoid meat produced in these ways, farmers, supermarkets and governments will be forced to change their policies.

But it's not all bad. Meat is an important part of our economy and an invaluable source of protein. Beef, in particular, is a great source of iron and omega-3 fatty acids. When I look at the ethical and health issues surrounding meat, two or three organic meat meals a week, with a good selection of nutritious vegetables, beans, lentils, wholegrains and fruit, feels about right. Let's not forget that although a good vegetarian diet with lots of beans, lentils, wholegrain, etc. is of course fantastically healthy, a diet full of processed foods such as fried vegetarian sausages, too much dairy and oily pastries, isn't. In fact, a vegetarian diet can be far higher in saturated fats, calories and sugars, and far lower in fibre, etc. than a meat-based diet.

Eating soya when you've been been diagnosed with cancer

Although studies still don't give us any clear guidance on eating soya-rich foods if you have been diagnosed with an oestrogen-dependent type of breast cancer, I would suggest staying away from soya as much as possible. A little isn't going to cause anything disastrous, I just mean that you shouldn't choose the soya-rich options on menus, or think about becoming vegan at this stage in your life. Sadly I think the possible downsides of creating an environment that could potentially encourage the growth of these tumour cells far outweighs any potential benefits you may glean from soya. If you're vegetarian this presents a practical hurdle, as so many vegetarian foods are soya-based, so try to focus on lentils, beans, nuts, seeds and grains like spelt and quinoa as good sources of protein, which are all delicious when cooked well.

Read more on:
▲ Pages 59–63

strained by the cancer and by the potent chemicals being put inside you, it's also very apt to look at the food hygiene issues I mention in the pregnancy section ▲, as the last thing you need is to develop a food-poisoning infection that will make you feel worse and interfere with your treatment. Intake of oily fish should be limited in pregnancy and for women of child bearing age, but this doesn't apply here, so if you fancy some smoked trout or salmon or a little smoked mackerel pâté you can have up to four 140g (5oz) portions in a week.

I would suggest that you think twice before you start downing the so-called 'supplement drinks' that are on sale in pharmacies for anyone who is experiencing poor appetite or nausea. These high-calorie, high-protein, high-fat drinks can have their role in a minority of situations, when nothing else suits or is available, but they're pretty sickly and can fill you up so that you're not able to eat a nourishing meal later on. If you could have a soup made with a good stock, with some thick Greek yoghurt added to it, served in a beautiful little bowl, this would feel far more normal and something all the family can share instead of sipping on a nutri-drink. I feel that we need to gain confidence in real food and how this can be tweaked to fit our cancer treatment.

You may find that nausea comes in waves and certain times of the day are less problematic for eating, so try to keep an open mind and capitalise on those times of the day when you don't feel so sick. We get set in our routines, but you may find that you need to have your evening meal earlier on or that you have five smaller meals instead of your usual three. If you keep a food and symptom diary ◆ as you're going along, this can help you work out how the spectrum of the different foods and nutrients is working out over a 24-hour period.

Read more on:
◆ Page 11
▲ Page 86

Cauliflower cheese, page 209

Remember, though, that your body can do with good supplies of as many of the key nutrient groups as possible, so if you can manage some fruits and vegetables and a few sources of protein as well as what appeals most – toast, pasta, etc. – then this is a real plus. You could find that cooked vegetables suit you more than raw ones, as they aggravate acid levels, but as long as you keep cooking time to a minimum you will still glean some useful vitamins such as vitamin C. In the case of beta-carotene, be reassured that the body is more easily able to absorb it from a cooked carrot than from a raw one – so don't worry that you're not getting much nourishment if all you fancy is cooked fruit and vegetables. Something simple such as a jacket potato stuffed with a little butter, salt and freshly ground black pepper may soothe and appeal.

If you don't feel like chomping your way through a steak or a piece of chicken, think about incorporating protein in something more appealing, such as a small portion of shepherd's pie, which contains all sorts of vegetables as well. Experiment with the topping, which could include cauliflower or carrots as well as the traditional potato. If you're feeling lousy and don't fancy a plate or bowl of anything, then a big mug of clear, consommé-style soup could be both comforting and nourishing.

You could also incorporate egg or nut milks ▲ into pancakes as they provide a little unobtrusive protein. If you can also manage it, a sliver of lean ham or smoked fish, or some pure fruit spread or sliced banana and a little butter on top can be especially nourishing and delicious. We so often just need ideas to get us out of the rut which chemotherapy and being labelled as ill tends to throw us into.

Sore mouth and swallowing difficulties

As with sickness, a sore mouth or an unpleasant taste are pretty common side-effects. One of the reasons why the mouth and the gut tend to be hit hard when we undergo many of the cancer treatments is that the drugs hit the cells, which rapidly divide, and this includes our gut (the skin and the hair being two other targets for a similar reason). As with sickness, discuss it with your doctor to see if your drugs can be tweaked, but if you find that your mouth is sore this can affect the type of foods you feel like eating. Sometimes a mouth can be more sore when it's dry, so drink plenty to keep it moist.

If hard or dry food is a no-go, try dishes like risotto, loosened with plenty of stock or something very saucy like cannelloni or lasagne made with plenty of rich tomato and meat sauce. Soup and noodle dishes can work too and if you use a good base stock and perhaps throw in some soft poached chicken or small prawns, you can have all the key nutrient groups in a delicious, comforting, easy-to-swallow meal.

You may find that softer breads work better, and are even easier without the crusts on. They are easiest to swallow when fresh with plenty of moist fillings inside, such as egg mayonnaise (made with ready-made mayo), cream cheese and very thinly sliced and peeled cucumber. Poached fish such as trout with mayonnaise or a little cream cheese are good too. Salt beef can be very soft, and if you add some thinly sliced tomatoes and a little mild mustard it can make a delicious sandwich.

Try to make soups as nourishing as possible by adding ingredients such as Greek yoghurt, crème fraîche or cream at the end, as this boosts the calorie content, while croutons can add interest if the soup feels too liquidy. One thing doctors worry about when we're undergoing cancer therapies is losing too much weight, as this can alter our blood work and disrupt our body's reaction to the invasive drugs and therapies. Try to keep this in mind and think about what you can add to dishes – olive oil, butter, cream and finely grated Pecorino or Parmesan cheese to puréed and mashed vegetables, for example, or a thick creamy custard made with full-fat milk to stewed fruit, served with a soft melt-in-your-mouth fine buttery biscuit. If porridge is your thing in the morning, make it with full-fat milk and add some cream and brown sugar or honey before serving. Putting a good layer of butter or nut butter on toast could make it easier and more enjoyable to eat, as well as higher in fat and therefore a more intense calorie hit.

Casseroles and tagines tend to produce soft textures and can be a good option if you add some little dumplings or serve them with gnocchi. Cooking meat for a long time, for example a slow-roasted shoulder of lamb, can render the meat ready to melt in the mouth ◆. With fish, the way you cook it can make a big difference, as can the size of the fish – bear in mind that the amount of time and effort you have to put into preparing foods can take the edge off your hunger, so you don't really want to be picking your way through small-boned, fresh sardines, especially if missing a bone could mean you catch what is already a sore mouth or throat. I'd go for larger, fleshier fish, where the bones are easier

Read more on:
◆ Pages 97–98

Pearled spelt, goat's cheese & chard risotto, page 203

to remove, and if you bake or poach them in stock, the flesh can be delicious. An obvious choice would be to make a fish pie, as the creamy sauce and soft, fluffy, buttery mashed potato often hits the spot. They can be made in small ramekins, enough for one or two to share so that one cooking effort can be turned into a few meals that you can freeze and use later, when you're not feeling up to cooking.

Sorbets, ice creams and frozen yoghurts need not be seen as treats but more of a necessity! The coolness can be soothing, but sometimes you may need to let them melt slightly, as anything extremely cold can cause more irritation. Sorbets can be more refreshing, but they're usually lower in calories than ice creams and frozen yoghurts (which, by the way, can be even higher in fat than ice creams). Small pots of sorbet, ready-made ice cream desserts and cold yoghurt or mousse au chocolat are worth keeping in your fridge, as they sure beat hospital food! Bear in mind that home-made ice cream sometimes contains raw egg, which can cause salmonella poisoning if your immune system is compromised, so watch out. Do take up offers of having food cooked for you, and let friends and relatives stock up your fridge and freezer, as it's one less thing for you to do. It can also be good for those around us to feel they're doing something helpful, healing and comforting.

Healthy heart

You probably don't need me to spell out how widespread and costly heart disease is – its effects on our day-to-day lives and our society are enormous. One of the most heartening (excuse the pun) headlines should be that we can in theory have a big role to play in reducing the incidence of cardiovascular disease, as most of the risk factors bar genetics are in our control. We often read about how smoking, high blood levels of the wrong kind of cholesterol and being inactive or overweight – particularly if we're storing fat around the middle ◆ – all increase our risk of developing heart disease, but so does having the less-talked-about type 2 diabetes ▲. There are other risk factors coming to light through research, including high levels of an amino acid called homocysteine, low birth weight, the presence of inflammatory markers and other immune system factors. It's early days for some of the researches to give us clear guidelines, but not for others: we do know that keeping our weight within the ideal range, not smoking, keeping active with a healthy blood pressure, and keeping our blood fats in

Read more on:
◆ Page 116
▲ Page 149

Chicken & chickpea burgers, page 212

check, will all make an enormous difference to the risk we place on our hearts and circulation.

I'm going to focus in this section on how, by eating certain foods, you can get your heart and blood vessels in good shape. The cholesterol story is pretty well documented – too much LDL cholesterol is bad and too little HDL cholesterol isn't the best either ◆. If you're unlucky enough to have already been diagnosed with heart disease, getting your diet in order is even more important. Not only can you help to prevent any further furring up of your arteries, but there is also some evidence to suggest that you could in fact help to reduce any damage that's already been done – so it's never too late to look at eating and living healthily.

Read more on:
◆ *Page 29*

Chicken soup, page 231

Getting the balance right

It's important to look at your diet and the way you're living, even if your doctor puts you on cholesterol-lowering drugs, as reducing your risk of heart disease isn't just about tackling one aspect. In eating and living well you help to reduce the likelihood of any cholesterol depositing in your blood vessels, as well as the chances of experiencing other risk factors such as high blood pressure. If you eat well you're far more likely to feel well and lose any excess weight you put on. I think men especially sometimes think all that matters is their cholesterol level, and for some taking a statin pill seems to be the way to fix the problem. It's more complex than that, but I hope this section inspires you to believe that eating for a healthy heart is easy and delicious, especially since the arrival on our supermarket shelves of great oils such as avocado, rapeseed and hempseed.

It's a good idea to try to get the ratio of the bad and the good sorts of cholesterol right because by eating well we can ensure a good balance: we want a high HDL and a low LDL level. Diet is incredibly important and shouldn't be a hardship or difficult to follow, as we now have such a vast array of produce at our fingertips, either in the supermarket, or if we use the Internet to source small suppliers. What we need to concentrate on is the Mediterranean diet (see below) as this will correct the balance of good and bad cholesterol and provide very useful antioxidants, which help reduce the likelihood of LDL hardening the arteries.

Concentrating on the Mediterranean diet

The Mediterranean diet – from Italy, Spain, France etc. – is what we typically call a diet based around lots (five-plus portions) of fresh fruits and vegetables every day. It incorporates a wonderful variety of colours and types, so we glean a good spectrum of vitamins and beneficial substances our hearts love. It's fine to have favourites and to go through phases when we buy a large amount of something because it's economical, or in season, but it's best not to get into a rut and have too much of any one type of fruit or vegetable all the time. Every fruit and vegetable has something in its favour: some have more vitamin C, others are higher in beta-carotene, another antioxidant, while others are better in the fibre stakes.

It's easy to get into the habit of always buying the same things, so if you're a little stuck in your ways get a few cookbooks out, or tap into websites and food magazines to target a few different fruits and vegetables. I get around the issue of not having too much of one particular fruit or vegetable by using my freezer a lot, not only to buy frozen vegetables like peas, broad beans and spinach, but also to freeze the vegetables I've grown when they're at their best. I make soups, vegetable sauces, casseroles, trays of roasted vegetables, as well as blanching crops like French and runner beans so that they're there in the freezer when I need them at some other time of the year. If you get into this habit you'll also have the advantage of knowing that you've picked your vegetables at their best and frozen them quickly (vitamin C and other vitamin and mineral levels don't diminish much in the freezer, so when you come to eat them they'll still be nutritious). This can also be a way to get the best out of the supermarket 'buy one get one free' offers: even making a large batch of tomato sauce and freezing it in usable quantities can be very economical in both money and time.

You're better off with vegetable rather than animal fats, which need to be kept to a minimum. Olive oil is the classic Mediterranean choice, but try rapeseed, hempseed, and avocado and nut oils, such as walnut oil, in dressings. They contain omega-3 fatty acids, which help to reduce your risk of heart disease even further. Unless you're underweight, use vegetable oil sparingly, in non-stick pans, and drizzle it, perhaps even using a sprayer to minimise the amount. There are as many calories in vegetable oil as there are in butter and it can lead to weight gain, which, especially round your waist, can lead to high blood pressure and heart disease, the last thing you need.

You could consider one of the butter-like spreads rich in plant stanols or sterols, which can reduce cholesterol levels, but I have to say I don't like the taste much. You need around 2g (2,000mg) of either stanols or sterols each day (the amount you'd get if you spread one of these margarines on four slices of bread) in order to lower cholesterol by about ten per cent over time. They need to be consumed regularly, but they aren't the only way to lower your risk of heart disease. Some people walk away from their doctor or supermarket thinking as long as they use spreads, drinks or yoghurts containing sterols their hearts will be fine. I don't recommend my

Read
more on:
◆ Page 29

Green olive &
parsley focaccia,
page 238

patients use them, as I think it's far better to look at being more creative with the food you're eating to achieve your healthy heart goal; but, this said, if you're looking for a few products to help improve your blood cholesterol balance, these are an option.

Although meat is lambasted as not being desirable on the menu if you have a high level of LDL cholesterol ◆ , a piece of lean meat is completely fine. Not only can it be pretty low in calories while being extremely satisfying, but lean meat also contains some monounsaturated fats, including the beneficial long-chain omega-3 fatty acids, and minerals such as iron and zinc. The poorer-quality fatty cuts need to be avoided, as they can deal you a very hefty dose of LDL-producing saturated fat – as also do the creamy sauces sometimes served alongside the meat. I think a good pattern to get into if you like lean red meat is to have it twice a week.

The rest of the time I'd focus more on oily fish – again a couple of times a week. They're a very good source of omega-3 fatty acids, which, although they don't have much of a direct impact on either LDL or HDL levels, have benefits that reduce your overall risk of heart disease. As with meat, you need to be clever with the way you eat them – making a smoked mackerel pâté with butter isn't the ideal way, as the saturated fat in the butter increases LDL, and the salt, which aggravates blood pressure, far outweigh the benefits of the oily fish.

For the rest of your week, go for meals based around chicken (well cooked and not too buttery), white fish, game, and lentils and beans for veggie days. Choose wholegrains such as porridge (which our hearts love, as oats are wonderfully rich in a special type of soluble fibre) and wholemeal bread.

Fatty liver

The image these two words conjure up is not pretty, and it can be worrying when you're told that your liver is too fatty, but the good news is that you can turn the situation around easily by eating and drinking well. Having a fatty liver is most likely down to having too much of a lesser-known type of fat in your blood, called triglyceride – although some people with high triglyceride levels also have too much LDL cholesterol, which requires a little refining of what you eat. High triglyceride levels can also be associated with carrying too much weight – luckily the type and style of eating you need to adopt when you have a fatty liver is compatible with losing weight, so you can hopefully get some good results on more than one level. Of course if you can bring down your weight, specifically the amount of body fat you're carrying, this helps to reduce your overall risk of developing hardened arteries and heart disease, as well as giving you all the other benefits of being lower in body fat. Sometimes a diagnosis of a fatty liver is just the impetus you need to make some good changes in how, what and when you eat.

Triglyceride levels

The first stage in reversing a fatty liver is to reduce your triglyceride levels, which in turn will help your liver to shed some of its fatty deposits. This process tends to take weeks, if not months, so we're looking at a change of lifestyle here, not a quick fix. Triglyceride is a type of blood fat that's aggravated not only by saturated animal fats – butter, cream cheese, fatty meats, lard, dripping, etc. – but also by vegetable fats, which is where the treatment for someone with a fatty liver differs from that for someone with a raised bad cholesterol level.

Our liver doesn't distinguish animal fat from vegetable fat, so if you need to reduce your triglyceride levels, make sure your total fat intake is lowered (setting oily fish aside for the moment, as the long-chain omega-3 fatty acids can be beneficial). This means keeping your intake of vegetable fats, oils, avocados, nuts, nut butters, nut oils, etc. down as well, though you don't need to avoid them completely, as food often needs a little oiliness to give it good flavours. A vinaigrette dressing on a salad or a drizzle of olive oil over a dish of pasta is completely fine, but there is no point in going along with the Mediterranean diet, which can be heavy on the olive oil, or spreading your toast with thick layers of peanut butter, thinking you're doing your liver a favour, as you're not. A little drizzle or a thin scraping are the descriptions to think of here, not lashings.

Read more on:
♦ Pages 17–18 & 95

Cashew nut butter, page 229

The reason I set oily fish apart from other animal fats is that they contain the good long-chain omega-3 fatty acids, which can help reduce blood triglyceride levels and therefore help your liver. Once they're past the childbearing age, women can eat up to four 140g (5oz) portions a week ♦ – but don't worry if you're not much of an oily fish fan, as just a couple of portions will give you sufficient omega oils to improve your blood-fat levels.

GI values

In addition to watching your fat intake, you need to watch the sweet stuff, as triglyceride levels are aggravated by high-GI foods. I can hear the sighs, but simply put, this means staying away from sugar, glucose, honey, sweet foods like biscuits, cakes, chocolate, fruit juices and ice creams. It also unfortunately means not overdoing the sweeter fruits and fruit juices, because although they contain some additional benefits such as antioxidants and fibre, too much high-GI fruit isn't good either. This means you need to steer clear of bananas, melons, raisins, grapes, dates, mangoes and pineapples. Instead, focus on citrus fruits such as oranges, clementines, satsumas and grapefruit, stone fruits such as apricots, plums and greengages, plus apples, pears, rhubarb and berries – they may not be exotic, but they're scrumptious. The trick for dealing with the fact that these fruits are slightly more tart is to cook them well – for instance, cooking rhubarb with an apple, a vanilla pod and some orange zest or star anise imparts lovely flavours that occupy your taste buds so that the tartness isn't so apparent. Roasting or chargrilling fruits also changes how tart they taste. On the vegetable front there are just a few to watch – baked and mashed potatoes, cooked carrots, squash and swede as they have a higher GI value too. All the others are good to include, so you should think bowls of steamed greens, ratatouille, big veggie soups and stuffed vegetables.

With fruit juices you have to be especially careful not to think that more is good, as unfortunately when fruit is changed into a juice some of the fibre is lost. You don't need to avoid juice, but you should have perhaps just a small glass every other day instead of the more common daily habit many seem to have got into since the arrival of ready-made smoothies. One way to make the drink last longer is to dilute it with a little water, or, if you're very thirsty, quench your thirst with water first.

Other good foods to eat are beans (borlotti, cannellini, kidney, black-eyed, haricot, etc.), lentils (ranging from the black or dark green Puy lentils to red and yellow and wholewheat pasta. And of course you can get spelt and other grain pastas, which, although they generally don't contain as much fibre as the whole durum wheat pasta, do have more fibre in than the white, so they're a good middle-ground to try. All these higher-fibred grains, beans and lentils are fantastic for helping to get a good triglyceride level.

When it comes to bread, since wholemeal bread very surprisingly has roughly the same high-GI value as white bread (wholegrain rye bread such as pumpernickel has one of the lowest GI values of the breads), I would suggest that you don't just choose bread according to its GI value – breads are generally best in their wholegrain form, be this the fluffy wholemeals or the darker, seedier, malty German-style wholegrains – as they provide fibre, B vitamins and other nutritional benefits. When it comes to your liver just watch that you don't eat too much of them. I think the superfood and positive nutritional labelling culture has led to a mentality that more is always better – but more cereal with added fibre or more wholegrain bread can lead to being overweight as well as having too fatty a liver. Less (that's good nutritional quality) is what I would call more here.

Seeing the results

If you make these sorts of changes to your diet as well as looking at how and what you're generally eating, you will most likely find that any excess weight will come off gradually and easily. If you reach your ideal weight and body-fat level you need to ensure that you don't keep losing it, as this isn't healthy either and can leave you depleted – so just check that you tuck into good-sized portions of nourishing foods and eat enough.

If you were of an ideal body weight and fat level (which is rare but not unheard of) when you were told you had a fatty liver, have a go at incorporating as many of these changes as possible, making sure you don't reduce your portion size. You could find that if you cut right down on fats and sugars you may find that your weight drops too low or you find yourself exhausted and ratty because your body is just not receiving enough of the good stuff, which includes calories. As I mentioned, this should be a lifestyle change, not something where you sort it out and then go back to your old ways, as the likelihood is that your liver will complain again in the future.

The only thing you may think it's a good idea to be pretty black and white about avoiding is alcohol. Since alcohol unfortunately aggravates a fatty liver, your doctor may want you to avoid it altogether for a while. Although people are generally told that a couple of glasses of red wine is a good health-protecting mantra, it appears now that we shouldn't put red wine up on a pedestal. You should treat it like any other alcoholic drink

Liver cleansing

If you want to consider complementary remedies, carrot and pomegranate juices are said to be good for the liver. Pomegranate juice provides some antioxidants and may also help reduce bad LDL cholesterol levels, while carrot juice has been used as a liver cleanser for centuries. If you like either of these, try having a small glass a few times a week – be aware, though, that pomegranate juice can be rather sweet, so is best diluted, and too much carrot juice can turn your skin orange! Others swear by taking milk thistle – the usual dose is up to 300mg three times a day.

and either have it in moderation or consider avoiding all alcohol until your triglyceride levels return to normal and your doctor gives the all-clear.

Diabetes

Diabetes is a life-long condition that, if not managed well, can lead to kidney damage, blindness and a higher risk of developing heart disease and stroke. Diabetics have too much glucose in their blood (which comes from digesting carbohydrate and is also produced by the liver) because their pancreas either: doesn't produce any insulin; doesn't produce enough insulin to help glucose enter the body's cells; or the insulin that it does produce doesn't work properly (known as insulin resistance).

Type 2 diabetes is the most common form and usually occurs when you hit middle age or in your older years. However, South Asian and black people are at greater risk and it can appear when they're much younger, although it is rather alarmingly also becoming more common in children and teenagers of all ethnicities. It does not usually require insulin for treatment (unlike type 1 diabetes), instead, patients must eat healthily and take drugs to help their system handle sugars more efficiently.

If you're diagnosed with type 2 diabetes, it's important to get to grips with your eating habits, as they can have a profound effect on how your body copes and how you feel. You don't need to resort to eating diabetic products (which can be unpleasant and expensive) as your eating style should be no more complicated, and just as delicious, as everyone else who follows a well balanced and nourishing diet. This can include some delicious cakes and biscuits, as long as you eat them in moderation (as everyone should) and make them as nutritious as possible by basing them on wholegrain ingredients such as wholemeal flour and fruits. This way you'll not only be enjoying some scrumptious cakes, but also taking in valuable fibre, vitamins and minerals, which, in combination, help your body stay and feel well.

If you're carrying too much body fat, then losing this healthily and steadily can have a very positive effect on your blood sugar levels. It's also particularly important to build a good exercise routine into your schedule as this will not only help you to lose weight, but will help the body maintain good blood sugar levels. Since having diabetes also increases the likelihood of developing heart disease, it's good to ensure you are eating the right types of fats as this will also help to reduce your risk.

Teenage Needs

This is a key age for experimentation, which as a parent, you can use to your advantage. As teenagers' interests begin to change you can introduce them to new foods and win their taste buds over to things they wouldn't previously touch (when they are hungry they'll eat anything). Often it is at this age that we start to become interested in cooking and begin to learn to cook for ourselves. This brings about a new understanding of food, which yields many positives as long as teenagers are taught the importance of a healthy diet and good-quality food.

This is a time when you are going to need your parenting skills more than ever. Teenagers may appear physically grown up – more than capable of looking after themselves in many ways – but actually they still require a lot of attention, time, support and of course love. You may have to find diplomatic ways of conveying all these things – they are not little children any more – but it is your job and not theirs to keep the lines of communication open. Nine times out of ten they may push you away, but the one time they don't it is absolutely vital you are there. It's a challenging time all round, but if you approach it with a positive outlook, the great thing is that you can instil healthy habits that will sustain your child throughout their life. When all lines of communication are down, sometimes being able to sit and eat together can be just what you need to open the channels up again – though this is not the time to harp on about the vegetables not being eaten. Let it go and relax – something in their stomach, even if it's a takeaway, even better if shared with you, even in silence, can be just what you need to draw a line in the sand.

Parenting teenagers

Pause for a moment and think about what being a teenager was like in your day: a melting-pot of hormones, emotions and body changes that played havoc with your confidence, mood and sense of wellbeing. Few people ever describe their adolescence as 'the best years of my life', and frankly it's no wonder. You may find the slamming doors, uncommunicative grunts and baffling language hard to deal with, but do have some sympathy. Teenagers today have it worse than we did in so many ways: more exams, which equals more stress; and more exposure to unrealistic 'perfect' body shapes, while fast food and excessive alcoholic intake play a huge part in teenage social life. Excess can lead to them gaining far too much weight and all the associated health and psychological problems. Let's not forget, too, that teenagers are inheriting a world which at times feels unsafe, confusing and pessimistic no matter how old you are – all in all, it's no wonder the teenage years are often not the easiest to work through.

A time for sensitivity

You probably don't need me to say this, as you'll know how sensitive you need to be around your teenager, but this is not the time for jokes about chunky thighs or spots – such comments are not only unkind, but positively destructive. The number of teenagers and older adults among my patients who can recite a remark by a parent as something that tipped them over the edge into an eating disorder is horrifyingly significant. There's a fine line to tread when knowing what to say about their body if they're either end of an ideal body weight. Of course it's your role as a parent to help them if they're gaining too much weight, but equally it's not good to focus on it, as that can cause their confidence to be dashed, leading them to either eat secretly, or lose all the excess weight and more, swinging right down into anorexic behaviour.

Some parents, especially mums, can be so fearful of their child becoming anorexic that they never talk about weight or eating issues – they think that if it's not discussed, their teenager won't think about it. But I don't think this helps – being able to talk with your child about any sensitivities they have and coming up with practical help to get them through it can be invaluable. The likelihood is that they will all be talking about it at school and see some of their friends sadly having big issues with disordered eating – be this anorexia, bulimia or being overweight. At least if you keep the lines of communication open you have a chance to put their minds at ease and to instil some common-sense, simple, what's-good-to-eat knowledge. Celeb-style magazines often spout utter nonsense about what celebrities supposedly eat and don't eat, and they also come up with copious amounts of pseudo-nutritional facts which can prey on your child's mind and get passed around their peer groups. If you're able to dismiss these by getting them to read this book and eat nourishing foods with you, you have a good chance of getting them through the teenage years unscathed by the mad disordered eating-world they're surrounded by.

This is not the time to start banging on about how you wish you were two stone lighter. Deal with that yourself quietly and without fuss. You also need to be aware that concerns over eating and body image aren't exclusive to females – society exerts many pressures on young men too. Gone are the days when a stocky man with a bit of a paunch was seen as a solid bet – models and fashion all provide a very different example of how young men feel they should look. Many want to be perfect, all muscley and six-pack-ridden, so be sensitive. It's a good idea to write down in a private notebook issues you don't want to pass on to your child, and keep referring to it.

The right foods

The adolescent years are physically dominated by the production of the sex hormones such as oestrogen, progesterone and testosterone, which bring about all sorts of physical and emotional changes. Little girls go from a child shape to the more curvaceous womanly shape that is defined by an increase in body fat levels, whereas boys start increasing their muscle mass and filling out – all of which requires teenagers to eat enough nourishing foods to enable the body to mature correctly. On a practical level, this doesn't mean you need to change the balance of the types of foods teenagers eat very much ◆. Boys don't need to start tucking into whole chickens or downing protein shakes, and neither do girls need to start increasing their fat intake – so long as they eat well, the body should take care of the changes. Really, you should think in terms of the teenage body just needing more of the types of nourishing foods they ate as children.

Read more on:
◆ Page 14

There are a couple of watch points for girls: if they're dieting or not eating much, and are restricting their fat and protein intake in particular, their menstrual cycle could be disrupted, which has the potential to affect their fertility and bone health in the future. Menstrual bleeding means that each month girls lose some iron, which you should try to replace by eating an iron-rich diet. Iron also provides a key role in cell replication, so it's essential for teenagers, both boys and girls, to eat enough to meet their growth needs. Sometimes, though not always, the body craves what it needs – in the case of red meat, you could find your teenager craving a lean steak, and this can be the case particularly with girls at different times of the month. Mind you, boys can eat large amounts of red meat too, and although they need to have enough to provide iron, it's important that the meat they eat is lean and good quality so that their intake of trans fats and saturated fat isn't too high.

Rapid growth, coupled with a fast lifestyle and poor dietary choices, can result in iron-deficiency anaemia, which can make you look and feel tired or breathless, experience poor concentration and affect mental and physical development in children and teenagers. Teenage girls are particularly at risk because their iron stores are depleted each month following their period, as are infants over the age of six months, menstruating or pregnant women, vegetarians and vegans, and people with conditions that affect absorption of food, e.g. IBS ◆.

Read more on:
◆ Pages 171–172

Weight problems

The teenagers I see as patients are often struggling with their weight – eating either too little or too much. Comfort-eating often signifies that their emotions are in turmoil, so if you can find a way to make sure they eat regularly, you can save them a great deal of unhappiness, both now and later on. You need to explain to them that what they do has a real impact on how their bodies will be in the future – a badly nourished body during the teenage years carries a greater risk of developing problems, such as osteoporosis and infertility. This can be a pretty compelling reason to help some girls click out of the notion of extreme underweight being seen as attractive. If you starve yourself during your teenage years, it may also have a pretty devastating effect on your metabolism as when you do begin eating normally again, the weight can pile on. I see many 40-something women who look back with huge regret at not being kinder to themselves when they were younger.

The best way to encourage teenagers to have a comfortable relationship with food is to eat with them as much as possible and teach them simple cooking skills. Don't nag, though, as the last thing food should become is a battleground. The aim is to try to get enough good food into their systems so they won't have the urge to binge. The secret lies in always having delicious and nutritious food available that takes only minutes to prepare.

Girls in particular often develop a phobia about sweet food, which they perceive as being fattening. You need to help them build up their confidence, introducing sweet dishes that are wholesome and healthy, such as carrot cake or date and walnut cake. It is important they learn that eating something sweet does not equate with their weight spiralling out of control.

Be sensitive to the fact that your daughter in particular may not want to eat stodgy dishes. I think it's completely counterproductive to try to get teenagers to eat food that you know makes them feel uncomfortable. If you insist on it you're going to have a battle on your hands – either then or, worse case scenario, if they eat it and then disappear off to the bathroom.

Dieting

Read
more on:
◆ Pages
160–161

Tomato & herb
salad,
page 220

Mothers in particular can worry that by explaining the calorific value of food to ours daughters, in a bid to help them prevent piling on the weight in later years, we are wilfully inflicting potential eating disorders upon them ◆. What absolute nonsense! We have a far greater problem in our westernised society with obesity than with anorexia or bulimia, and if you enable your child to know how to be able to select healthy foods, this is ideal – what food contains and how much or little they need to eat are among the most important life skills you can teach them.

If your child is unhappy about gaining extra weight, don't tell them they look fine – take their concerns seriously. Plenty of teenagers put on so-called puppy fat and it is the fat, not the losing of it, that can lead to a negative body image. In addition, being overweight can lead to children being horribly bullied. When that happens, they can suffer all kinds of psychological problems, from low self-esteem to feeling suicidal. So if they come to you asking for help, make sure you provide it, rather than leave them struggling on their own. However, it is also important to encourage them to have a realistic expectation of what their body can look like – what was your own body shape like at this age? Help them achieve a look that gives them confidence, but which is also as healthy as possible.

Sensible, controlled dieting can be an excellent opportunity for you and your child to talk about food and introduce good habits for the future. Show them that it is possible to control weight through delicious, nutritious dishes, rather than extreme behaviour. Help them by not keeping items such as crisps and biscuits at the front of the cupboard although there may be members of the household who don't have a problem with their weight, so you don't want to make them completely off the radar. Try to replace the space they filled with snacks such as dried fruit, unsalted nuts, crispbreads, etc. It also helps to have a fridge full of light foods such as raw vegetables, soup, stewed fruits and natural yoghurt that they can have if they've come home ravenous and need something small.

As an eating pattern, place the emphasis on plenty of vegetables and salads, with moderate amounts of protein, such as chicken and fish. Don't ban any food – just encourage moderation. Bread, pasta, potatoes and rice can all be enjoyed if eaten in sensible quantities. Even chocolate is fine if you buy good quality, 70 or 85 per cent, which is virtually impossible to eat in huge quantities even though it's delicious. Stay positive about food and don't chastise children if they fall off the wagon. It is a fine line to tread, but if you can instil a basic love and appreciation of food, rather than allowing it to become the enemy, you will have more chance of them developing bodies they are happy and comfortable with for the rest of their lives.

Taking time over meals

In an ideal world we would eat with our children every evening, but life is not that perfect. Eat with them when you can – at least once or twice a week – or the second-best scenario is to sit with them and talk while they eat. Food is a social activity and one we usually enjoy more when there are other people around. Eating on our own is quite lonely, which is why so many people sit in front of the television, but try to discourage this at least some of the time – food is something that needs concentration in order to fully appreciate it. Teenagers who eat while they're watching TV, wandering around or on the phone are far more likely to become overweight and have problems with digestion. The gut needs to be still to deal with food, so try to encourage them to sit down, even for a snack – it takes nothing more medicinal than this.

Teenagers often rush their food, so again encourage them to eat slowly, as this will help the body recognise when it is satisfied. As with all stages in life, their meals should include a good balance of foods from the key groups ♦. If a meal is too light it will leave them complaining of being hungry later on – you may think a simple salad is all you need at lunchtime, but their rapidly maturing bodies need something more substantial. Equally, something that is very sweet, fatty and low in fibre and protein – typically fast-food junk – will satiate them only for a short time. People get addicted

Read more on:
♦ Page 14

Ten tips for helping your teenager lose weight

- Hydration plays a big part, so get them to drink at least two and a half litres (10 cups) of water throughout the day – weak squash (no added sugar) also helps.

- Encourage them to only eat at mealtimes – if they need a snack they should sit and eat it slowly, concentrating on what they're eating.

- Keep to three meals a day plus fruit snacks between meal. Insist on them eating breakfast, even if it's just a banana and yoghurt or a smoothie (home-made, ideally). This will improve their moods and energy and make them less inclined to snack mid-morning.

- Cook nourishing meals for the whole family to share; don't isolate your teenager and make them feel different because they're on a diet that no one else is happy to eat.

- Don't keep crisps, biscuits, chocolates or fizzy drinks in the house. Suggest that once a week they can enjoy a treat outside the home, say a cake at a coffee shop.

- Make sure the fridge and cupboards are stocked with plenty of simple nourishing foods, so that hunger doesn't lead to snacking on something junky.

- Teach them five quick dishes they can make for themselves – even a toasted sandwich made with wholemeal bread is a good made-in-a-minute option.

- Choose activities that expend energy. Sports are an obvious option, but don't forget boxing, martial arts and dancing, as these are fun and good for burning calories. It's amazing how short walks and less time in the car, can help and exercise gets your body to manufacture mood-enhancing endorphins.

- Try not to eat in fast-food restaurants. There's nothing wrong with a simple pizza Margarita and a salad with the dressing on the side (so you can control how much you add), but watch Caesar and blue cheese dressings, de luxe salads with croutons or bacon bits, etc., as they're all high in fat and sometimes sugar, and you've probably read that many fast-food salads contain far higher calorie values than a simple burger made with good-quality lean red meat, especially without cheese.

- If you feel it will help, set some targets and non-food rewards – losing about a kilo (two pounds) a week is roughly what to expect, although we're all different. It may be that simply noticing clothes getting looser week by week rather than actually weighing seems the better strategy.

to fast food and want to eat more and more of it because of the lack of satisfaction as well as the high fat and salt content.

What's in the cupboard?

In reality, a lot of the time your teenager will want to 'graze' or grab a quick snack before bolting out the door again and will rarely sit down for a proper meal. The trick as a parent is to ensure that there is good food available when we want it, however, the last thing we need is for our house to be seen as a juice and salad bar with nothing but boring health food fodder around. This will only lead to teenagers staying well clear and eating out all the time, as they crave something more substantial – and this may be junk and processed foods, which you'd rather they avoid. With sensitive girls, in particular, you don't want to give the impression that they should only be eating salads and low-fat yoghurts, but on the other hand it's not a good idea to stock cupboards with copious amounts of crisps, sweet drinks and chocolate bars. You need to provide a good selection – some treats like good-quality chocolate and unsalted nuts and dried fruits, but also plenty of foods that provide stomach-filling goodness as a snack or a more substantial meal put together in no more than ten minutes.

When it comes to main meals, make sure you have a few good staples such as pasta (ideally wholemeal, but white is still good), which teenagers can boil and stir a dollop of pesto or tomato sauce into – show them how to make a quick snack so that they have the confidence to do so. Another good storecupboard staple is good jumbo porridge oats that they can grab in the morning with a chopped banana, a handful of frozen berries or a dollop of apple sauce. I've got into the habit of soaking the oats in milk overnight in the fridge, which makes not only a good porridge but also a base for adding seeds, nuts and dried fruits (you can soak the oats in apple juice if you prefer, and stir in a dollop of creamy yoghurt along with the nuts and fruits). Keep a stock of fish fingers in the freezer, plus individual packs of wholemeal bread rolls and pitta breads that can quickly be made up into a fish 'burger'. Eggs are another essential standby – fried, boiled, poached or in an omelette, they make easy, nutritious dishes that cost little time or money.

It's good to get teenagers into the habit of eating properly, but if all this feels like too much effort and they're flying out the door, then whip them up a smoothie with fruit and oatmeal that can be devoured in less than two minutes.

It's also worth remembering that teenagers often travel as a group. If you want to monitor whether your own son or daughter is eating a nutritious diet, the clever thing to do is make sure yours is the house known for always having food available. As well as keeping the cupboard well stocked, keep dishes in the freezer that will satisfy the hungry hordes. There are many simple things – a simple tomato, meat or vegetable sauce – that they can dip into or that you could turn into something such as a sausage bake, lasagne, cottage pie, or a batch of meatballs; then all they need to do is microwave it and serve with a warmed pitta bread, dollop of relish and a few salad leaves for a meal in minutes. It's also good to have a few lighter dishes for the girls, such as chicken casseroles and vegetable stews. Don't forget to have some sweet things around – carrot cake, date and walnut muffins, fruit crumbles, sorbets, etc. – as the more you encourage teenagers to eat at home, the less chance there is of them eating in fast-food outlets or skipping meals altogether.

Teach them to cook!

Teach your children to cook from as early an age as possible. You'll be surprised how interested many teenagers are in cooking (thanks to the many TV food programmes and inspirational celebrity chefs) and it may become something they excel at. Even if they're not keen on learning much, anyone can be taught how to boil pasta, bake potatoes, whip up scrambled eggs or heat up baked beans. If you know they love a particular dish of yours, teach them to cook it. Let them see that preparing food is fun, enjoyable and much more than a chore. I think the most useful piece of kitchen equipment to have with a teenager around is a hand-held blender to rustle up quick soups and smoothies. Remember that as they learn to cook they will probably ruin every frying pan you own and leave the kitchen in a terrible mess.

When teenagers exhibit worrying eating patterns, I think cooking has a role to play in enabling them to build up a healthier relationship with food. If they're worried about their weight, they can so often think sauces are packed with calories, or that you put lots of fat in dishes when really there isn't much at all. Magazines come out with such nonsense about food that it can be a nightmare for someone sensitive. If teenagers cook (shopping is also a good thing to get them to do) they can take control of food in a more constructive way – once they're involved in the food preparation they can put together something lighter that they're happy with but the rest of the family can still join in with eating. This helps take the spotlight off their sensitivities and keeps the lines of communication open. If you serve

Tandoori chicken, page 213

something rich and overwhelmingly stodgy, you will only exacerbate their fear and they will most likely refuse to eat with you, resulting in all sorts of chaos and unhappiness in the home. But if they are involved in cooking the food themselves, it takes the pressure off you – so let them cook and let them feel proud of doing something helpful and pleasing.

Eating disorders

I know I'm going to challenge the traditional views of how to treat what we can loosely term disordered eating. Let me just say here that I'm not talking about the very underweight, anorexic teenagers who need specialist help, I'm talking about the far larger group of teenagers who struggle with eating and body weight. The traditional way of treating teenagers with eating disorders is to force them to eat regular high-calorie meals in order to get them to put on weight. Simply put – and I'm not saying all clinics are like this but the majority of them seem to be – if you don't eat the food and put on weight you don't earn rewards such as seeing relatives, getting your own music, etc. It's my experience that this therapy doesn't work, as all that happens is that they are forced to eat, gain weight, and then, as is highly likely, struggle so much with what they're meant to eat and how their body is feeling that they will get into a mess again and lose far too much weight as a result.

Although everyone is different, and a key element in helping your child with an eating problem is to get good psychological help if you feel it's gone beyond what I call worried eating, I think it's far better to allow them to eat lighter foods. They might not have as much, say, carbohydrate (which many don't seem to like to eat in large amounts), but I think it's much more important for them to eat regular meals containing nourishing ingredients, such as roast chicken with a salad that has a few beans or lentils thrown into it. If you offer light meals your teenager will feel comfortable about eating and you can add bulk to it for other family members by serving extra pasta or bread in a separate bowl. If you are going out for a meal, choose a place where your child can order sushi or salad rather than everything-with-chips.

Being aware about what they are eating does not necessarily equate to an eating disorder. The teenage years are tough emotionally and physically, and if your child is sensitive and conscious about food they need to know they can talk to you about issues and not either get their head bitten off or be forced to eat what you think they should be eating. The more laid-back you are, the sooner they're likely to click out of controlling their weight and join in with the rest of the family. Experimentation is a normal part of the teenage years, and food is often a part of that. If you respect this and offer healthy nutritious meals in moderate portions, there's no reason why it should escalate into anything serious.

People with eating disorders are usually not comfortable around any food at all. Having a preference for the low-fat variety simply indicates a quite normal teenage preoccupation with how their body looks. The warning signs are: that they don't want to eat with you; that they say they've had a meal, but you never see them eating one;

that they blatantly skip meals; that they won't even eat something you know they love; that it seems that they say are not hungry all the time; that their weight has changed significantly in either direction over a couple of months; that they have rituals around how they eat; that they are particularly body-sensitive; that they over-exercise; and that they start to cut themselves off from the rest of the family. In addition, they may start to wear dark-coloured clothes that appear to shroud them, which can be a sign that they are feeling ashamed of their body.

If your teenager fits any part of this description, do not panic. Do not immediately march them down to the doctor or arrange for them to be admitted to a specialist centre as you could be adding fuel to the fire. If you can keep your child eating with you, no matter how small an amount they consume, you have a chance to pull the situation back from the brink. Do not offer high-calorie, high-fat dishes in a bid to 'build them up' – they are more likely to be tempted by a food they perceive as non-fattening. Don't stand over them insisting they eat or turn food into a battle of wills between you and them and don't let them see how anxious you are. If you are co-parenting, it is important that the two of you work together on a cohesive course of action, agreeing to discuss it only in private. If you do show support and a great deal of

common sense, it is possible that you will be able to gently wean your teenager off the food-phobic path. Only when you have exhausted all possibility of recovering the situation yourself – and if their weight is clearly plummeting – should you seek professional help for anorexia.

Bulimia (classically bingeing on food and then purging through self-induced vomiting) can be a much harder problem to spot. Look out for a very slim body with a face that looks puffy and bloated – the latter can be brought about through fluid retention caused by repeatedly making oneself sick. Bulimics may not have the outward signs to trigger concern, but inside they are doing a lot of damage to their bodies. This can result in ulceration, indigestion and even breathing difficulties from stomach acids leaking into the oesophagus – serious hardcore bulimia can result in electrolyte imbalances that can be extremely serious. If your child asks for help and it's not happening that often, you may want to see if you can sort it out as a family. Help them to break the routine by first listing the foods they do feel comfortable about eating, no matter how few this is. As previously mentioned, it is important to help them eat regular, light meals and end the dangerous cycle to which bulimia can lead.

(Note: boys are just as capable of developing a serious eating disorder as girls.)

Teenage moods

We all remember these, don't we? The slamming doors, the you-don't-understand-me mantra, the sudden onset of tears ... Well, I'm not promising miracles, but you will be delighted to know that there are plenty of practical ways that you can help to deal with those adolescent mood swings.

Depression and anger

By this, I don't mean actual clinical depression, but the sudden lows teenagers encounter, almost as though they're plummeting through the floor. Sudden anger is often a sign of depression, which manifests itself in teenagers prone to tantrums.

Read more on:
◆ Pages 170–171

Maya's chocolate brownies, page 245

The first thing you should check, with girls in particular, is whether they are iron-deficient, as depression can be one of the first signs of anaemia. Coeliac disease ◆ is an intolerance to gluten and can be a lesser-known culprit, as it diminishes the gut's ability to absorb iron and other key nutrients. Both anaemia and coeliac disease can affect sleep, which in turn can lead to depression.

You should also consider their refined sugar intake, as it is my experience that too much can cause an instant high followed by a dreaded crash, which plays havoc with teenage moods. It's worth checking to see if teenagers are eating or drinking lots of sweet stuff and be aware that it seems to have its most powerful effect when they consume it on an empty stomach. Having said this, the highest GI foods, which raise blood sugar levels, are in fact, not that sweet-tasting – white rice, white bread, bran flakes etc. – so you may be better off encouraging them to eat the wholegrain varieties.

Is your teenagers' caffeine consumption too high? Are they having too many high-energy, high-sugar drinks and not enough water? Being dehydrated can itself be a mood dampener – often we feel low and moody but within minutes of drinking a glass of water the mood can lift. Are they actually eating enough? Remember how crotchety they were as small children when they were hungry? Well, there is no difference now they are twice the size – and in fact those growing bodies require more food than ever. The hormonal changes that are going on can also change their appetite, which explains why girls can have the munchies at certain points in their menstrual cycle and boys can have an enormous appetite when their increase in testosterone production calls them to start bulking up. Skipping breakfast, smoking and too little exercise can also be important factors in affecting moods.

Broken heart

The melancholic pain of a broken heart is different from depression. Love is a powerful force, no matter how old you are, so don't make light of the pain your child is suffering. This is not the time to say there are 'plenty more fish in the sea.' Teenagers can feel absolutely invalided by the hurt they are going through so you should also heed any warning signs of negative body image – the idea that 'he wouldn't have dumped me if my thighs weren't so enormous.' Broken hearts can lead to a severe loss of confidence, which, in rare cases can spiral into an eating disorder ◆.

Read more on: ◆ Pages 160–161 ▲ Page 167

Spicy fish casserole, 216

Going off food is often a sign of heartbreak, as the very thought of eating can make the broken-hearted feel nauseous. It is important to get some food into their system, as the nausea will only get worse on an empty stomach and their bodies will quickly become depleted of vital nutrients. Even if it is only a soup or a smoothie, it will do them the world of good. Girls in particular often crave sweetness when they are unhappy. Rather than see them munching sadly through sweets and chocolate bars, introduce some delicious home-made treats, such as chocolate mousse or comforting chocolate brownies. Give them plenty of love and sympathy, but don't overtly criticise the lost boyfriend or girlfriend – they may be back together in a week or two!

Anxiety

Teenagers today have good reason to be anxious: they are stressed out with too many exams, are bombarded with 'ideal' bodies through the media and are faced with an increasingly uncertain world. It is your responsibility to help them through their worries and fears. Much of this centres on the same advice given for depression (see above): plenty of water, not too much caffeine, regular nourishing meals, moderate alcohol and nicotine intake and some light exercise. Good sleep is also a huge factor ▲.

A high-fibre breakfast such as porridge, muesli, fruit, yoghurt or wholemeal toast followed by a protein-rich food such as eggs, beans or smoked salmon is a good option if they've got a big exam session ahead. Surprisingly, couscous made with nuts and dried fruits can be good too – I think it's the combination of easy eating and the sweetness of the dried fruits, without liquid, that makes it a good stomach-settler. If they are too nervous or feel too sick to eat, try to get them to eat just a couple of pieces of fresh fruit – bananas have a particularly good stomach-settling effect. A piece of fruit or a fruit smoothie – ready- or home-made – is another good stopgap.

Too much caffeine can exacerbate anxiety, so although a warming cup can be good to wake them up, watch that they don't have too much.

Try to keep them off energy-stimulating drinks, as they can make them feel wired and unable to concentrate on the task in hand. If you find you have a very nervous teenager and think that a cup of something soothing and calming is what's needed, try giving them a herbal tea – the ones that traditionally have been used to calm include chamomile, catnip, bergamot and lemon balm. More potent sedative teas include skullcap, blue vervain, valerian and hops, which you could try in the evening to help them wind down ◆.

Read more on:
◆ Pages 35–36
▲ Pages 146–148
● Page 11

Make sure they are drinking enough water and encourage them to hold off on sweet or fizzy drinks, chocolate, sweets, biscuits and other sugary snacks – fresh fruit, dried fruit, unsalted nuts, smoothies, yoghurts and soup are far more beneficial. At night, starchy foods such as wholegrain rice, pasta, potatoes and bread can make them feel more relaxed and prone to a better night's sleep.

Panic attacks are bad news no matter how old you are, but can be absolutely terrifying for teenagers. The adrenaline rush causes a racing heart, sweating and anxiety and is often followed by feeling completely shattered. The first thing to ban is caffeine, although interestingly, research shows that people who drink a lot caffeine become tolerant to it, so it is less likely to make them more anxious. It's the teenagers (and adults) who are particularly sensitive to it, or suddenly increase their caffeine intake, who may notice a difference. Alcohol and certain illegal drugs such as cannabis can also feed anxiety, so try to discourage your teenager from wild nights out.

Look at how generally well balanced their diet is. If you eat regular, nutritious meals you are far less likely to suffer from anxiety than someone overdoing the fast-food, high-GI type ▲. Try instead to go for medium- to low-GI foods, which include most fruits (except bananas and dried fruits), raw vegetables, pasta (white or wholemeal), porridge, rye bread and rice (brown or white).

Teenage bodies

Some teenagers (especially boys) can be extremely skinny, so you are lulled into thinking that they're not eating enough or are avoiding junk food when in fact, this is often not entirely true. They are very good at filling their bodies with unhealthy food without anyone realising or any weight gain. They can still do themselves some damage, so as a parent, you need to watch what they're eating. Perhaps you could occasionally ask them to keep a food diary ● or do it as a family so that you don't alienate them or put them under any pressure.

Menstruation

When girls start menstruating their bodies can go through all sorts of physical and emotional changes as a result of the alterations in sexual hormones such as oestrogen, progesterone and testosterone. Mood swings can rock from one extreme to the other and teenage girls can suffer from very bad menstrual cramps, become bloated and uncomfortable, and develop spots. Forget all the nonsense sold to us in tampon adverts, that imply that you should carry on as normal through your period. The fact is that any young woman should be allowed to feel under the weather, because periods can be debilitating. Nature is a powerful force; one theory as to why women feel so exhausted before their period is that it is the last time in the month you have the potential to get pregnant. By slowing you down, nature makes it more likely a man will catch you and mate with you! Many young women need some extra TLC at this time, so keep a diary of your daughter's menstrual cycle and be prepared to be extra nurturing if she is unfortunate enough to suffer with bad period pains, bloating and moodiness.

Read more on:
◆ Pages 171–172
▲ Pages 160–161
● Page 106

Pain and bloating are enough to make any young woman feel negative about her body, particularly when they are so out of her own control. IBS symptoms are ◆ common during menstruation, because the gut becomes sensitive to changes in oestrogen and progesterone levels. For some girls, menstrual discomfort and mood swings can lead to a scenario where they try to stop being women by starving themselves, a dangerous move that can lead them to developing an eating disorder ▲. If you talk to your daughter about how she is feeling and show concern and sympathy, she is less likely to become fearful about what she is going through.

Happily, there are also practical steps you can take to help her through it. Perhaps one of the most significant nutritional challenges is the fact that starting menstrual bleeding is the first time girls are confronted by a regular loss of iron. You need to up her iron levels, both immediately before menstruation and during it. She may not be keen on the idea of eating liver – the traditional old wives' cure – but she can also take in iron through lean steak, eggs, dried apricots and green-leaf vegetables, such as kale, dark Savoy cabbage, rocket and spinach. Try to keep her off strong tea and coffee, especially when eating iron-rich food, as they diminish iron absorption.

Bloating is another down side of menstruation and one that figure-conscious teenagers can find particularly upsetting. Some foods, such as cauliflower, Jerusalem artichokes and onions produce a lot of wind ●, so may be better left off the menu. Cooked vegetables are also generally kinder to the gut than raw ones. Fluid retention can also be aggravated by too much salt and not enough potassium, so prepare dishes based around herbs and lemon juice, rather than salt and pickles.

Water is essential (fluid retention is not caused by water), and a diuretic tea such as dandelion may help. Smoothies are also easy to digest, and again, ones that are potassium-enriched are ideal, such as banana and orange or grapefruit and raspberry.

Boys' bodies

While girls are coping with periods, boys are having a similarly confusing time with an overload of testosterone. Testosterone isn't just a male-only hormone – women produce it too – and the same applies to the female hormones such as oestrogen, which boys also manufacture. Boys often overproduce oestrogen during puberty, which can give them slightly larger breasts and even cellulite ●, which usually disappears. The hormonal cocktail that surges into action during puberty causes boys' bodies to undergo similarly rapid changes in shape, albeit less rounded and more about building muscle than women. The hormonal shifts can also change their skin, making it more prone to spots, oiliness, and of course smelliness. And need I mention the moods and the changes in energy levels? One minute they're perfectly happy to be out clubbing all night and the next they won't move from their bed all day!

Read more on:
♦ Page 45

We often talk about how some girls are preoccupied with their body shape and the way their body is changing into that of a woman, but we shouldn't forget that this time of change can be equally challenging and upsetting for boys. Boys often worry about not growing up as fast as their peers (or growing too fast) and height and bulk start to become very important. Some boys feel shy about developing facial hair and a deeper voice, while for others developing a six-pack can become a preoccupation – we only need look at advertising campaigns and men's magazines to see that there is huge social pressure for boys and men to have the perfect body.

Boys can get confused with what to eat – so you need to step in here. They often think they need to start drinking protein shakes and eating whole chickens in order to bulk up, but this isn't the case – it's the combination of good regular exercise, both aerobic and non-aerobic. Running, swimming, cycling and longer-lasting lower endurance exercise alongside muscle development and weight training will increase chances of having the flat-board stomach and chest that many aspire to! Note – a gym workout does not mean a huge increase in calorie intake. You may feel ravenous afterwards but you'll not be doing your body any favours if you double the amount of food you eat.

Sleep

At any age, sleep is important. Unfortunately, teenagers often slip into bad sleep patterns, going to bed too late and then feeling exhausted during the day. Iron deficiency can also cause poor sleep, so it can be something that girls suffer from during menstruation. Lack of sleep can also lead to terrible mood swings and poor performance at school. Caffeine is very often a culprit in exaggerating all of this, so watch teenagers' consumption of high-energy drinks, tea, coffee and chocolate. If they want a sweet 'fix', try to provide it with fresh fruit or home-baked flapjacks, which are packed full of oats, carrot cake made with wholemeal flour etc. These are far more gentle on the body and less likely to unsettle blood sugar levels, which can be disruptive to sleep patterns.

Try to introduce comforting soporific foods, such as bananas, wholegrain rice or pasta, in the evening, which fill the stomach and are also very relaxing. Starchy, warm dishes are the perfect inducement for sleep but avoid dishes with lots of spices in them, because some people find them to be quite energising and may irritate the gut, which can also disrupt sleep. You only need to sniff some chilli powder to see what effect it has on your heart rate and how powerful it can be!

Milky drinks have a fantastic lulling effect, but remember that milk contains a natural sugar called lactose, which is slowly released so you don't necessarily need to add anything else to it. Chocolate, which contains a caffeine-like substance called theobromine, can be a stimulant, but if that is what appeals, make your own by melting a couple of squares of 70 per cent cocoa chocolate into the milk, as this is good quality with very little sugar in it. Plain milk with a touch of honey is sweet and comforting, particularly for people who don't like the natural sweetness of milk. Most hot chocolates are fine – whatever your teenagers fancy, serve it in a nice big mug and let them really savour the experience. Look out for night-time milk – literally milk taken from cows that are milked at night – as this contains a higher amount of the sleep-inducing chemical, melatonin.

Hair

The appearance of our hair is crucial to our self-esteem, so hair loss can be upsetting, particularly for teenagers. If hair is thinning, take your teenager to the doctor to check for anaemia or low ferritin levels (the body's store of iron). Are they eating enough? If protein levels are low, hair will be affected. A low-fat diet will also have an impact because the follicles need sufficient oils – if for no other reason, this can be a good motivator for getting your son or daughter to be less strict with themselves. There are other complaints that can affect hair, ranging from digestive ones, such as Crohn's disease, to skin conditions such as eczema. The contraceptive pill can also have an impact and lacklustre hair can be a sign of psychological problems, such as bullying at school, so always heed such warning signs.

If your child wants to eat well to achieve a healthy mane of hair, the secret lies in plenty of iron-rich foods, such as good-quality red meat, game or offal. One or two good-quality red meat meals each week should be enough to keep iron levels healthy. If this is a teenage turn-off, encourage them to eat plenty of green, leafy vegetables, such as spinach, dark green Savoy cabbage, curly kale, broccoli and asparagus. Egg yolks, pulses (including baked beans) and fortified cereals are also beneficial, but try to choose a healthy, low-sugar, low-fat version if possible. Proteins have the double benefit of meeting the hair follicles' high requirement for amino acids.

Read more on:
◆ Pages 92–96

Many children decide to become vegetarian ◆ in their teenage years, so you need to make sure that they eat a balanced diet. An extreme vegetarian or poor diet can also cause hair loss later in life. If your child is a strict vegetarian or vegan, you may need to seek professional help, because it can be hard to increase ferritin stores to a sufficient level without the help of supplements. Iron supplements are notorious for their negative effect on the gut so you need to make sure you consult a doctor or nutritionist. In order to assist the body to absorb iron, you need to increase the intake of foods rich in vitamin C: berries, mangoes, kiwis, oranges, citron pressé and smoothies. Serve an iron-rich meal with a small glass of orange juice or offer fruit for dessert. Don't allow coffee, tea or cocoa drinks during or after such a meal, because the polypherols block the body's absorption of iron. Also watch out for green teas, because although their polypherols are generally seen as a good thing, they can also block iron absorption, so it's best to drink them between rather than with meals.

Skin

Spotty skin is the cause of much teenage angst, so it might be that your child can be persuaded to eat more healthily on the grounds of vanity if nothing else. It is a myth that chocolate causes spots and that dairy products block the pores. What the skin does need is plenty of hydration and enough replenishing nutrients, such as zinc, vitamin C and iron. Antioxidants and omega-3 fatty acids are also essential, and can be taken through a good combination of vegetables, juices and oily fish. Oily fish are also a rich supplier of protein, essential for growth and development, which are after all occurring at a breakneck speed at this age.

If your teenager is vegetarian or vegan, I'd suggest they take a vegetarian omega-3 supplement to cover their needs. This will take the pressure off, and means they can just enjoy eating seeds and nuts as part of their general diet without thinking they've got to consume a certain amount in order to meet their omega-3 requirement. You also need to make sure that your teenager's diet is high in fresh fruits and vegetables, that they drink plenty of water and generally eat a well-balanced diet ◆.

*Read
more on:*
◆ *Page 14*

*Cashew
nut butter,
page 229*

Food intolerances – fact and myths

The incessant bombardment of nonsense food stories in the press means that many teenagers convince themselves they are intolerant to something. I see many people in my practice who think that their symptoms, such as bloating, wind, an uncomfortable gut or skin conditions, are down to intolerance of a food such as wheat, when in fact the problem within their body comes purely and simply from their lifestyle: not enough good, regular meals, eating the wrong things, too little sleep, too much alcohol or nicotine. So instead of rushing to exclude foods, one of the best things you can do is teach teenagers about the impact of food on their gut.

This is particularly important if their diet isn't that well balanced in the first place – if they're fussy eaters, the last thing you need is for them to be even more limited in their food choice. This can cause all sorts of spin-off problems, such as being worried about food and the way their body looks, as well as leading to physical problems such as lack of energy and depression. For girls, restricted eating can prevent their body from maturing, so try to get them to eat a well-balanced diet for a few weeks and see if the symptoms disappear. If they don't, then you can of course explore whether specific foods need to be targeted.

Candida

As deeply uncomfortable as the symptoms can be, there is a lot of nonsense around about the effects of too much Candida albicans in the system, and teenagers may start to believe that they should be following an anti-candida diet. It is true that sometimes, if you have had to take a lot of antibiotics, you can end up with an overgrowth of candida (which can cause thrush).

However, the idea that certain foods will do the same is irrational: all food is eventually broken down into glucose, which is the only fuel we can use in our bodies. The idea of cutting out sugar, yeast, mushrooms and alcohol in order to kill candida bacteria is really pseudo-science.

Sometimes symptoms such as headaches, bloating and tiredness do in fact improve on an anti-candida diet, but that is simply because this diet is healthier than usual – cutting out sugars, fast food and alcohol never did anyone any harm. If your teenager wants to follow such a diet, take it as an opportunity to explore some healthy eating together and to talk about what the body really needs in order to stay healthy. Try to dissuade them from following any diet that involves fasting or excluding certain food groups; as they need a balanced diet for general health, and there is a danger they will build up a bad relationship with food and end up more moody and depressed than when they started. They can also become low on valuable nutrients, which can affect the look of their skin and hair.

Read more on:
◆ Pages 104–105

Lemon polenta cake, page 252

When it comes to the problems caused by too many antibiotics, introducing probiotics and prebiotics ◆ can help reinstate the bacterial balance within the colon, which can help ease problems such as wind and bloating. You can offer these either as a supplement or in something tasty such as Greek-style yoghurt.

Coeliac disease

Coeliac disease affects one in 100 people and is caused by a reaction to various proteins found in wheat, rye, barley and oats, including gluten. These proteins damage the part of the small intestine that enables the body to absorb food properly. The disease runs in families and particularly affects people from the Punjab region of India, Pakistan, the Middle East and North Africa. It is also common among people with type 1 (insulin-dependent) diabetes, autoimmune thyroid disease, osteoporosis, ulcerative colitis and epilepsy.

Diarrhoea and malnutrition are the most common symptoms of coeliac disease. Children may fail to gain weight and grow properly, while adults may find they lose weight. Malabsorption of essential proteins can also leave people feeling tired and weak, because of anaemia caused by iron or folate deficiency. Other possible problems include mouth ulcers, vomiting, abdominal pain, itchy rashes on the elbows and knees, infertility, osteoporosis and bowel cancer. Some people who are intolerant to wheat may have undiagnosed coeliac disease so it is important to consult a doctor. Although there is no cure, it can be controlled by carefully following a gluten-free diet and it is important to understand which foods are gluten-free and which contain wheat, barley and rye. Many can be

Read more on:
◆ Page 124

Wild rice salad, page 222

successfully substituted and recipe books and gluten-free foods are readily available. A diet rich in calcium and vitamin D and regular weight-bearing exercise are also essential to help prevent osteoporosis from developing ♦.

Irritable Bowel Syndrome (IBS)

This is an umbrella term for a number of symptoms, the most common being: bloating, gripes, constipation, diarrhoea, wind, nausea or a bad taste in the mouth. Although any serious symptom should be checked with a doctor, more often than not these sorts of digestive symptoms are signs that an aspect of their lifestyle needs to be tweaked and this is not necessarily just based around what they eat. It's good to see if there are emotional reasons for their gut being upset before rushing them to see a gastroenterologist or embracing some sort of food exclusion diet at home – it might be an indication that your teenager is having a tough time at school or college, for example, as emotional upset can sometimes manifest itself physically in this way. Sometimes teenagers just won't articulate why they're struggling with something, as life can feel pretty complicated, and this affects the way their body deals with food – anxiety and stress can increase acid secretion in the stomach, which can change the way that food is dealt with. It can make us more tense and less able to go to the toilet, so we can get into a troublesome cycle of constipation or the opposite, having to rush to the toilet when we're worried. Of course, being preoccupied with woes can make us skip meals, eat things on the run, crave foods that aren't the best to eat – so all in all it's not surprising that IBS can start at this age. (Menstruation can also trigger IBS-type symptoms.)

A good place to start with nutrition is to explain to your teenager that the food they eat has a very real effect. If they go to the pub and then for a Chinese takeaway at midnight, they will suffer the consequences the next day. Of course you can't expect them to always eat healthily, but do try to help them understand the link between the foods they eat and how they feel. The gut is a muscle and it needs oxygen in order to work. If we eat and then dash off somewhere, the oxygen will be pumped to our legs, not the gut – and the gut may start to complain. Try to get teenagers to cut down on alcohol and nicotine, drink enough water and eat small, well-balanced, nourishing meals three times a day.

In addition to eating well, you could increase the level of prebiotics and probiotics in their diet – this means looking into natural or Greek-style yoghurt, as this is a natural probiotic if it contains live cultures, which survive passage through the GI tract. Eating live probiotic natural yoghurt helps them to build up good levels of bacteria, which can alleviate some

Read
more on:
◆ Pages
104–105
▲ Page 11
● Pages
90–91

Pearled spelt,
goat's cheese
& chard risotto,
page 203

symptoms of IBS ◆. Prunes (and figs) are natural laxatives, delicious with probiotic yoghurt as a good quick breakfast or with something like a no-added-sugar muesli-type better-for-you breakfast cereal. The combination of natural yoghurt, fruit and high-fibre cereal can often provide a good remedy for painful constipation.

If bloating is a problem, encourage teenagers to keep a food and symptom diary ▲, recording everything they eat and drink for a week. From this you will be able to see if they're eating a healthy diet or whether a simple thing like eating more fruit and a high-fibre cereal or wholemeal bread instead of white, could suit them better ●. You may like to see if they prefer a diet that's not heavily wheat-based – which can so easily be the case when they're huge cereal fans, have a sandwich lunch and then eat pasta in the evening. Maybe a tweak or two, changing to, say, rice or rice noodles or even a spelt or other cereal-grained pasta, might just address the imbalance. We so often get stuck in a routine, but if we can think outside the box and be a touch more adventurous with what we eat, IBS can become a thing of the past.

A note on spelt

Spelt is a distant cousin of wheat and has a lot of its versatility making delicious bread, pasta, cereals, etc. However, some people find (for reasons largely unknown, as research studies are still in their infancy) that spelt seems to suit their digestive system better than wheat. The structure of the protein in the spelt is different – gluten being more brittle and differently absorbed by the gut – and if you look at well-sourced and well-produced brands (which are usually organic and don't come into contact with contaminants), you may find that your body prefers spelt-based products. Spelt comes in the form of pearled spelt, which you can make into a risotto, as flour for all sorts of delicious bread, pastries and biscuits, and also as pasta. You can also buy pastas, biscuits and other traditional products made with buckwheat, oats and rice, so check these out too.

Glandular fever

Glandular fever, which is caused by the Epstein-Barr virus, can be a horribly debilitating illness common to this age group. Affecting people in numerous ways, from aching joints and depression to exhaustion, it can develop into ME and chronic fatigue syndrome. It is important, therefore, to support the immune system with a healthy nourishing diet rich in antioxidants found mainly in fruits and vegetables. Zinc and selenium also benefit the immune system, so encourage teenagers to eat foods such as unsalted nuts, red meat, chicken, shellfish, pulses and wholegrains.

Although it's tempting for teenagers to just grab something when they're feeling lousy, it's best if they avoid the pattern of grabbing a quick fix of energy, and then slipping back into sleep or inactivity. Not only does the crash that follows undermine the body's ability to get stronger, but if this is all you eat then you run the risk of becoming depleted in essential vitamins, minerals and other key recovery nutrients such as proteins and complex carbs. Structure can also be useful when it comes to activity, as research has shown that if you include a daily programme of exercise and activity, as opposed to just lying around with little to distinguish your days from nights, the recovery time from illnesses such as Epstein-Barr virus and ME shortens.

If they are suffering from a very sore strep throat (which often coincides with the Epstein-Barr virus), you should look to dishes that will slip down with relative ease, such as fruit sorbets, soups, soufflés and risottos.

Coughs and colds

Colds and sniffles are much less serious adolescent complaints, but can affect the moods and behaviour of your teenager. Dairy products are not responsible, as many believe, for causing blocked sinuses – and to deplete the body of calcium at this age is a mistake. The answer is to strengthen the body's immune system through nourishing soups and the like. Honey and lemon is a classic and effective remedy for cold symptoms as it has powerful soothing and healing effects. I usually have some when I'm feeling under the weather or going down with a cold (or indeed want to try to stop myself catching one of Maya's). Whatever the illness, hydration is very important: aim to drink two to two and a half litres (10 cups) of water a day, staggered sensibly, with just the occasional cup of tea or coffee.

Spicy fish casserole, page 216

Looking After the Older Generation

As we enter our late 60s and early 70s, our bodies, along with the way we eat and the lifestyle we lead, tend to change significantly. There can be huge differences between a 70-year-old who's sprightly and continues to lead a very active life, and someone who due to physical or mental health problems needs a lot of care. For the vast majority, reaching this stage of life brings new nutrition- and food-related challenges.

Eating well or feeding someone nourishing food can be such a pleasure, and something we can hopefully have some control over. However, this can be more difficult in hospitals and care institutions as they don't seem to be able to get it right at all, in my opinion. Why shouldn't this stage in our lives incorporate eating delicious food we know is good for us?

As I've dotted around the various ages through this book I've found myself with even more difficulties in making generalisations, but I've identified some concerns that are good starting and discussion points. I hope they will inspire you to look at other sections of the book to see how you can tackle and work your way around them.

Look after yourself

Some of the challenges that arise as we reach old age are because old habits die hard. The temptation is to think that we can eat whatever we want and continue a similar lifestyle – after all, that's what we've always done. However, both our body's ability to deal with the food we eat and all other aspects of our lifestyle begin to change and our diets need to reflect that. We are also more at risk of developing certain diseases such as heart disease and stroke. But help is at hand, as we have far more sophisticated health screening and diagnostic tests now, so that we can look at things such as cholesterol levels and see whether our blood vessels are furring up, which is information that wasn't available in the past. We also know so much more about how making changes to our diet can have a really positive effect on our health before problems begin to appear and it feels like it's too late to do anything about it.

Although I don't want to imply that life should be focused entirely around food, it's especially important when you reach this stage of your life not to let things go when considering what you eat. You need to maintain interest in your body, as the difference between looking and feeling well, and being healthy on the inside can be strongly influenced by the foods you eat. You may find that frequent health niggles that start to appear at this age, such as constipation, poor energy levels, heart disease and diabetes can be made far more manageable by eating the right foods and caring for yourself. If you're looking after someone in this age group, food will enable you to give them so much pleasure and can be a great healer.

Sadly it's far too easy to fall through the cracks of the modern-day health system, and illnesses that need treating can be misdiagnosed or missed altogether. Even if you are lucky enough to be under the care of a good doctor or nurse, get back in touch with them if you find that your appetite starts going off, you're losing weight or notice any other changes in your eating habits. It's always best to catch weight loss early than to get into real difficulties when your appetite has gone and other symptoms arise as a result of not eating enough. Some drugs adversely affect appetite, so keep in regular contact with your doctor and discuss changing to an alternative if you think it could be more appropriate.

We often take weight loss and lack of appetite far too lightly, and many institutions don't prioritise eating nourishing meals. We should do far more to turn the situation around, rather than prescribing supplement drinks as if they're the answer to everything. Life should be more about eating nourishing, scrumptious food, and even more so when we're older.

Vegetables

Read
more on:
♦ Pages
106–108
▲ Pages
32–33

Cauliflower
cheese,
page 209

Vegetables are one of the most important groups of foods to focus on throughout our lives, but particularly as we get older, as they offer so many nutritional benefits, not least fibre. Lack of fibre leads to constipation ♦ and can mean that we don't get enough or any satisfaction from the meals we eat. This can lead to us eating too much of the higher-calorie fatty and sugary foods, which ultimately ups the risk of gaining too much weight with further consequences. Our body is at a stage when it could do without being put under too much weight as we carry the excess load.

One of the problems, looking at the practices in institutions and hospitals and at some older people's cooking habits, is that the vegetables that they eat are generally over cooked and not at all delicious or nutritious. If we overcook vegetables we lose most, if not all, of the vitamin C, and although there will still be some fibre our levels of essential vitamins can be too low. Lack of vitamin C means our immune system won't be receiving as much help as it could do with, and can compromise our ability to heal leaving us vulnerable to infections. Lack of vitamin C also reduces our body's ability to absorb iron, which we need a plentiful supply of throughout our lives. If we don't eat much red meat, we need to give our body a helping hand in absorbing iron from other iron-rich foods such as eggs, green leafy vegetables, lentils and beans ▲.

There is a case for using the freezer well when it comes to practical ways to boost our vegetable intake, as frozen vegetables – spinach, broad beans, peas, etc. – preserve their nutrient content and can be a good source of vitamin C, especially if cooked lightly, and are also fantastic for fibre. We can stock up the freezer and just use what we need rather than leave unused ones to rot in the vegetable rack. Tinned vegetables can often be disappointing, rather mushy and bland, but improved canning technology over the last few years that there are a few good exceptions: tinned sweetcorn, garden peas and asparagus spears tend to be fine, as can spinach and artichoke hearts. An omelette with peas and finely chopped prosciutto or streaky bacon can make a quick scrumptious meal, and throwing peas or sweetcorn into a ready-made pasta sauce stirred into pasta, along with pesto, or soup can be another easy way to up vegetable intake.

You can also buy pretty good soup nowadays, both tinned ones and fresh in pouches and cartons, with a good vegetable content (and often lower in terms of salt and sugar than the chilled soups). And of course it's a good idea to stock the freezer with individual portions of vegetable pasta sauces, soups, ratatouille, tagines and vegetable casseroles, if you're looking after someone. You don't lose any of the fibre or vitamins and minerals by blending a soup either, so if swallowing is an issue, a blended soup can be a great source of vegetables.

Vegetable juices are a fantastic way to glean vitamin C, folate and fibre. Make them fresh at home, using a juicer, or buy ready-made juices such as beetroot and apple or apple and rhubarb.

Keeping things moving

Read
more on:
◆ Pages
30–32
▲ Page 94

Not being active tends to slow down the way the lower part of your gut works and you may suffer from constipation, in which case you could find that you need to increase your fibre ◆ and water intake; doing gentle exercise such as yoga, walking or swimming can help to get things moving. Some medication can also have a constipating effect, so discuss this with your doctor – it could be that changing your drugs (codeine, for example, can be dire at bunging you up) could help ease things too. The most common constipation remedy to be handed out is lactulose, which can have its place, but it can also aggravate the bloated feeling – it's very sweet, and I think it's much better to see if you can get your gut moving by tweaking your diet.

Make sure that your diet includes lots of fibre-rich foods such as wholegrain bread, brown rice, quinoa, spelt, oats and cereals, plus fruits, vegetables, beans and lentils ▲, but you also need to keep your fluid intake up by drinking plenty of water. There are a couple of herbal teas renowned for getting the gut moving – those made from tamarind, dandelion or yellow dock, and infusions made by steeping fresh root ginger or four to five senna pods in 150ml (2/3 cup) of hot water (or you could try senna tablets from health food shops and pharmacies).

Being active helps the gut to move – even walking or yoga or swimming, something not too stressful on the heart or any other part of your body, can help to kick-start the gut into working better. Exercise can also help to reduce stress and anxiety levels, which can be contributing factors to constipation.

If you still have a problem with constipation, your doctor may prescribe a laxative, but don't be surprised if you find yourself feeling more bloated – this can be an uncomfortable side-effect and is the last thing your sore, constipated gut needs. If your constipation isn't too bad, or if you prefer to see if you can tackle it without taking laxatives, it could be worth trying to boost your intake of the naturally laxative-effecting fruits such as prunes, figs and apples. Sometimes just a few glasses of prune juice (which I suggest making up from prune juice concentrate), wholemeal toast spread with prune spread, or some stewed apple and rhubarb, can get the problem sorted quickly.

Drinking enough water

As we get older our ability to recognise when we need to be drinking more water or fluid decreases, and many people find that the less they drink the less they want to drink. Some care homes and hospitals don't want their elderly patients to drink much because of the practical issues of continence that this can trigger. I find this atrocious, as lack of fluid can cause all sorts of health problems: not least, it can make you feel shattered, fed up, constipated and can affect your concentration. Some care homes have their heating on quite high, and while residents may not be sweating, they can still lose a lot of water this way. Whatever the reason, we need to keep our fluid intake around two and a half litres (10 cups) a day.

Read more on:
◆ *Pages 38–40*
▲ *Pages 33–36*

As you know, I'm a huge fan of water – it's the most hydrating of fluids, meaning that you will glean the maximum hydrating properties from drinking it. If cordial makes the water more appetising, a glass or two a day can be a good way to up your water intake ◆. Tea and coffee have a mild diuretic effect (you lose a little bit of the water you've taken in as it stimulates your kidneys to get rid of it), but there is nothing wrong with a few cups of tea or coffee a day contributing towards this amount either. There is a lot of good to be gleaned from drinking tea ▲, but you should watch that you're not too generous with the sugar. The only liquid which has a dramatic diuretic effect is alcohol, so this shouldn't be seen as part of your two and a half litres (10 cups) a day target. If you don't have any contraindications for drinking alcohol, such as pancreatitis or being on certain medication, a few units a week can be pleasurable. And a little glass of something before a meal can be a good aperitif – especially useful if your appetite is off.

Rhubarb

Rhubarb is high in fibre, vitamin C, folate and beta-carotene, and is especially yummy when cooked with the juice of an orange or a little apple juice. Although spring tends to be the time when the majority of rhubarb hits the shops, and the more greenish-tinged rhubarb I grow pops up from May through to October. You can find force-grown rhubarb in the depths of winter but it tends to be more pink in colour and less tannic in taste, and therefore has a more delicate hit which may suit your palate better. Rhubarb can easily be cooked or blanched and frozen.

Butter

Many of us are big butter fans, but we shouldn't see it as being the only and the best source of fat, or use it in large quantities. Fats of all sorts contain a lot of calories, and when we were younger and more active, our body was probably able to justify a buttery slice of toast or portion of vegetables. As we get older, however, we tend to become more sedentary and our metabolic rates lower (unless we're very unwell), so if we're not careful too much butter can increase our weight and also our levels of LDL cholesterol, which can ultimately lead to heart disease.

Read
more on:
◆ Page 29
▲ Page 149

I don't want to say that butter should be banned altogether, but if you've been told by your doctor that your LDL cholesterol level is too high ◆ cutting down on butter can be one way to help bring it back down to a safe level. We do all need some fat in our diet to help us absorb fat-soluble vitamins and stop us from losing body fat, which is a good insulator and cushioning under our skin, so replace saturated fats with some other vegetable-based mono- or polyunsaturated fats. Try olive, rapeseed or avocado oil, or perhaps choose an olive oil based spread for your sandwiches, even if you are adamant that toast doesn't taste the same without butter. Every step you can take to ensure that you're not eating too much saturated fat is welcome.

Sugar

While a delicious sable biscuit or melt-in-your-mouth ginger nut with a cup of tea or a small portion of apple crumble with custard or a crème caramel after a meal can be part of our day, if we were to keep a record of how much sweet stuff we consume the amount might be higher than we'd expect. As part of our culture, we consider giving people gifts of sweet foods, such as a box of chocolates or truffles, to be one of the best ways to show we care about them. However, if we're not careful and we eat too much, we can hit problems when our refined sugar intake goes too high – for one thing, we increase the risk of tooth decay. Preserving our teeth and gum health is incredibly important, and sweet drinks, biscuits, etc., combined with poor oral hygiene, can conspire against us maintaining a healthy set of teeth and gums. If we have a small appetite, drinking too much sweet tea and nibbling on too many biscuits can make it far less likely that we'll be able to eat a nourishing meal later.

Read
more on:
◆ Pages
182–187

Poached
rhubarb &
blueberries,
page 241

Too much sweet food can pile on the weight too, which increases our risk of developing diabetes ▲ and heart disease, and can aggravate joint problems such as arthritis ◆. If we're carrying too much weight, getting around and exercising is far more difficult, so all in all it's a good idea to see if we can watch the amount of sweet foods and drinks we consume. There are so many delicious ways to enjoy sweet foods but at the same time reduce to the effects of having too much. The best scenario is if we can get our sweet hit from fresh fruits, perhaps a delicious orange or a slice of apple cake made with wholemeal flour, and in that way introduce some other health benefits such as fibre. If you can stick to three meals a day, with, say, a piece of fresh fruit as a between-meal snack, this is a good way to ensure that your body receives a good balance of the essential nutrients.

If you're having problems with your teeth that are affecting your ability to eat fresh fruits with tough skin, one solution is to peel or cook them. I cook Bramley apples in a large pot with frozen raspberries and poach peaches, nectarines and plums, then either freeze them in smaller portions or keep them in the fridge to dip into as a base for puddings or simply warmed up with a dollop of yoghurt. The only thing you need to bear in mind is that you won't receive as high a vitamin C hit from fruit when it's cooked, but it still provides a good source of fibre and other nutrients such as potassium and some folate. Do discuss any dental problems you're having with your dentist, as it may be that something can be done to make eating fruit easier and you don't need to suffer in silence.

Avoid getting low in vital nutrients

As we get older our body tends to become less efficient at absorbing or manufacturing nutrients; for instance, the skin isn't as good as it used to be at manufacturing vitamin D, so if we're not spending much time in the sun our vitamin D level can be worryingly low. This is why we are encouraged to take a 10mcg (400 IU) vitamin D supplement. But research also shows that older people can lack enough iron, calcium, B vitamins such as folate, and zinc – a lesser-known mineral which we need for a strong immune system and to maintain a healthy appetite.

Mass-produced food is notorious for being devoid of much nutrition, and is often not that appetising when it arrives. If you're a relative or friend of someone who's having to rely on institutionalised food, you could try to improve their nutritional status. It may be that as well as a vitamin D supplement, a more general vitamin and mineral supplement could help make up a few of the essentials, but discuss this with a doctor to ensure that it doesn't interfere with any medication they're taking.

Reduce the risk of food poisoning

When we're young and fighting fit it can be easy to get through a bout of food-poisoning, but when we're older it can be far more serious and in some cases, life threatening. We need to avoid foods we know carry a greater risk, such as runny eggs, soft cheeses, especially if they're

Avoid grazing

Just as large meals can put you off eating well, so can being a constant nibbler, as the nibbles usually end up being high in fat, salt and sugar and lower your appetite for nourishing meals. While constant nibbling on biscuits, nuts, sweets, etc. can do this, so can sipping on the supplement drinks often prescribed by doctors when appetites are poor.

Read
more on:
◆ Pages
59–63

unpasteurised, and pâtés ◆. We also need to be particularly careful with keeping foods well wrapped, fresh and stored well. This is where a freezer and a microwave can be useful, as they can reduce the length of time that food is sitting around and potentially growing food-poisoning bugs. As long as food is defrosted and cooked well, it can be a very practical answer. Flasks are great for soup, risotto, pasta, casseroles, vegetable curry, dahl, ratatouille and one of Maya's favourite school lunches, cauliflower cheese, if you need to cook something in the morning or early afternoon and you want it to be warm enough to eat later on.

Arthritis

The majority of people with arthritis, whether it's rheumatoid, osteoarthritis or gout, wonder if their diet might be either the cause or the cure of their joint problems. It's a big area of interest, not least because there are lots of supplements that promise to be the best thing for our joints, either in preventing arthritis or, if we already have it, in making a difference to the way it affects us. Cod liver oil and glucosamine are two of the most popular supplements, with green-lipped mussels and turmeric being more recent headline grabbers. As well as this, it has already been suggested that if we avoid acid-producing foods such as oranges and red meat, or have a daily dose of apple cider vinegar, our joints will love us.

Yet some doctors completely dismiss the notion that a diet or supplement will make any difference, and some can make you feel as though there isn't anything we can do to help ourselves other than lose weight. This is a shame, because I've found that we can make a significant difference to our symptoms and our overall health. We also need to bear in mind that when we go through a particularly rough time with arthritis, especially rheumatoid arthritis, we can lose a lot of weight quickly and all of a sudden look and feel much older.

Osteoarthritis and rheumatoid arthritis

Studies show, and indeed it seems to be widely considered, that diet can have a bigger impact on rheumatoid arthritis than the more common type – osteoarthritis. However, I'm going to deal with the latter first, because we are more likely to suffer from it in old age.

Osteoarthritis (OA) is a degenerative condition that develops when the cartilage around our joints, especially weight-bearing joints such as the knees and hips, wears away and new bone tissue grows beneath. This prevents the joints from moving as smoothly as they should, causes painful inflammation and over time, the joints may become distorted, causing further discomfort as muscles become strained and nerves get trapped. The main risk factors for developing OA are getting older, having a genetic predisposition to it, trauma or injury to a joint, and sometimes repetitive activity (which is the case with professional sports people) can make the joints become arthritic. Carrying too much weight is a strong risk factor, especially for developing OA in the knee – the joint which seems to suffer most from excess weight strain.

Of course a big problem resulting from osteoarthritis is that because the pain discourages movement, we don't feel like exercising even more, so unless we change our diet the weight can start piling on. This puts an even greater strain on the joints, particularly the knees, and up goes the inflammation and the pain. Interestingly, the link which exists between being overweight and having OA of the knee can be easily understood, as the less weight the knee has to support the less strain put on the joint, but the link that studies have found with being overweight and suffering from OA is far more complex than simply being mechanical. It's thought that being overweight and carrying too much body fat has an effect on blood fats and on hormones such as oestrogen which may explain the link which exists between OA and a greater risk of developing heart disease.

Whatever the subtleties physiologically, if you're carrying too much weight the first and most important thing to do is to try to bring your weight down sensibly: a couple of pounds (1kg) a week is a good rate. You need to do this healthily, as the last thing you need is to go on any sort of crash nutrient-depleted diet that will leave you feeling weak and ill. Sometimes doctors can be too forceful in their 'go away and lose weight' tactics, and you can feel bullied into going on a crash diet, but this isn't the answer – it's possible to sustainably lose weight by eating well without exacerbating any of your other symptoms. I think that one of the reasons why some people give up trying to lose weight is because they go on a diet that's so strict that it leaves them feeling weak and even more awful than they did before. It's interesting that if you're not overweight in the first place you have a lower risk of developing OA, but even if you have already been diagnosed, any shift in weight, however small, should help to make some of your symptoms better.

When it comes to the specifics as to what your diet should look like now that you have osteoarthritis, the main parameters should be the same as for anyone else your age. The more intricate links that have been found between specific foods and symptoms of arthritis seem to be connected with rheumatoid arthritis (a complex inflammatory condition that affects both young and older people). However, some people with osteoarthritis do seem to find that certain foods upset them or ease their discomfort, so although the evidence for the following areas of nutritional strategies is far stronger with rheumatoid arthritis, you may find something that could help you, whichever type of arthritis you have.

Read more on:
♦ Pages 143–145
▲ Pages 11
● Pages 17–18 & 95

Roast mackerel with potatoes & thyme, page 215

The overall diet can be best summarised by Mediterranean food – fruits, vegetables, oily fish being a few of the things to enjoy ♦. Most arthritis sufferers say that they can't eat too many oranges, tomatoes or other acid-producing foods as they make their joints feel worse. Interestingly, there is no hard scientific evidence to support cutting out any specific food, but rather than dismiss it completely I think it's worth keeping a food and symptom diary for a fortnight or so ▲. At the end of that time you can see if there is any relationship between what you eat and drink and how your joints and the rest of you feels.

My theory is that as long as you eat an overall healthy diet, you may just find that taking down the amount of specific foods or indeed leaving something out helps. If you feel better eating white instead of red meat, for example, this is fine, but my big word of caution here is that your diet should be healthy overall and full of nourishing foods. You need to watch out if you're cutting out fresh fruits, as these can be one of your richest source of vitamin C, if not the richest. Vitamin C is an essential vitamin for helping our body repair cuts and pressure sores and recover from illnesses – so it's important on every front to keep your fruit and vegetables up to the five-a-day target.

We don't understand exactly why, but diet rich in the long-chain omega-3 fatty acids found in oily fish ● stimulates the body to produce substances that can sometimes dampen the inflammatory response and alleviate arthritic pain. Although it has to be said that the evidence for long-chain omega-3 fatty acids being helpful is largely shown with rheumatoid arthritis, sometimes people with osteoarthritis experience some relief too. Since there is evidence to show that vitamin D (in which oily fish are wonderfully high) is also important in helping to relieve and slow down the progression of osteoarthritis, I recommend that it's good to ensure oily fish are a big part of your diet. Another option for increasing your long-chain omega-3 fatty acid intake would be to take a fish oil supplement, as this may help to reduce inflammation – you need one containing a total of 500–750mg of the fish oils EPA and DHA. Cod liver oil, although one of the most widely used supplements taken by OA sufferers, hasn't been shown to fare well, and even though some people swear by avocado and soy bean, again the studies don't give us much evidence for the benefits in taking them.

Getting back to your diet and the types of fat you eat, I'd strongly recommend that you choose monounsaturated fats as your main source of fat, as these are largely regarded as being neutral when it comes to inflammation (unlike the omega-6-rich oils – sunflower, safflower and corn oils – which are best kept down in your diet). Rheumatoid arthritis can increase your risk of heart disease, so choosing a diet based around a small amount of monounsaturated fat will also help you protect your heart.

Another common supplement is glucosamine (an amino acid sugar), but again there is confusion here as the industrial studies show them to be advantageous while independent ones don't. But some people swear by glucosamine, and some studies have shown that if taken regularly over several years it can be effective in increasing the rate at which cartilage is able to repair itself. The usual dose is 1–2g (1,000–2,000mg) per day. You may see glucosamine supplements that contain chondroitin (another component of cartilage), and although studies have cast doubt on whether these supplements, whether taken individually, or combined, actually show convincing results, my view is that if you find they do provide some relief, since there isn't any harm in taking them and there is little traditional medicine-wise which offers miracles, then I wouldn't stop taking them.

Gruesome gout

Unlike most forms of arthritis, gout tends not to last very long. It's an extremely painful inflammation that usually only affects one site – most often the joint at the base of the big toe, which some people describe as being so excruciatingly painful that it's as if someone has rammed a red hot poker into it. It seems to be more common in middle-aged or older men, and especially among those who love rich food although I'm seeing more and more women with hot, swollen, painful toes. There is, however, also a strong genetic link.

The inflammation of gout is caused by the release of crystals of monosodium urate monohydrate, which usually comes from the natural product of metabolism, uric acid. Sometimes this is caused by a build up of unwanted uric acid in the body, but a diet which is rich in purines (see below) can also increase levels of uric acid and trigger gout. There is a saying that 'the associates of gout are the associates of plenty', but more specifically, as well as not too much of the rich stuff, you should look to watching the amount of purine-rich food you eat. Keeping away from these as a general rule can reduce the likelihood that a gout attack will painfully spring itself upon you – it could also stop the first signs of gout (if you're in tune enough with your body to notice when perhaps the joint is feeling different, or indeed if your doctor has advised you that your uric acid level has come back high in a blood test) and prevent an attack from occurring.

The foods richest in purines and therefore best avoided or kept to a minimum include game, offal and meat extracts such as stock cubes, pâtés, sausages, meat pies and yeast extract (Marmite). Those red meat lovers among you may well be relieved to know that lean cuts of red beef, lamb and pork, as well as poultry, are slightly lower in purines, so are fine for you to eat in moderation. It's game and offal that can get you into the most trouble.

When we talk about oily fish, it's usually in a positive way, i.e. these are good for the joints, since they're rich in the long-chain omega-3 fatty acids. But unfortunately if you either have a genetic predisposition to gout or find that your diet is otherwise high in purines you also need to be very mindful that mackerel, sardines and herrings are purine-rich. Sadly anchovies, sprats, whitebait, and shellfish such as crab and prawns, are also high in purines, so I would suggest that if gout is on your radar you either look to taking an omega-3 supplement or stick to salmon and fresh tuna (which have lower levels of purines). More generally on the fish front, white and oily fish (salmon and fresh tuna, mentioned above) are great to eat, but too much smoked food such as smoked salmon, pickled herrings and rollmops isn't good for gout.

You could also look to include some of the vegetarian sources of omega-3 fatty acids, including hemp, walnut and linseed (flaxseed) oils – use these oils in salad dressings or as alternatives for frying or drizzling over vegetables. You could also sprinkle linseeds and walnuts (also good for your heart and blood pressure) on wholegrain cereals such as unsweetened muesli and porridge. However, unfortunately the types of omega-3 fatty acid you find in foods other than oily fish aren't of the long-chain variety, so I'd see using some of these oils and nuts as an added bonus, not as your main omega-3 fatty acid source ◆. Be aware

Read more on:
◆ Pages 17–18 & 95

Butternut squash & red lentil dahl, page 204

that too much oil of any sort will up your calorie intake, which may not be a good thing.

Finally, as if I haven't been enough of a killjoy already, and although they're usually seen as great nutritious foods, you may find that if you're particularly predisposed to gout, steering clear of dried fruits, peas, asparagus, cauliflower, spinach, lentils, mushrooms and mycoprotein (Quorn) could be just what your body needs to get its uric acid levels down. Wholegrain bread and cereals are good generally, but you need to avoid wheatgerm (generally bought as a single cereal in health food stores) and bran. Watch out for the deluxe mueslis, as they can be packed with dried fruits, which may just aggravate your gout.

Alcohol has been firmly associated with gout and historically, we can trace a link back to port and Madeira being the worst gout-triggering drinks. This was probably because they used to sweeten these alcoholic tipples with lead shot, chronic low-grade lead poisoning being a risk factor for gout. But nowadays, when port and Madeira are less commonly quaffed, we know that alcohol of any sort doesn't help gout, and indeed beer drinkers can be some of the hardest hit. You'll probably be warned off all alcohol if you're mid-attack, but afterwards drinking plenty of water alongside your alcohol can help to flush it out of your system and make it less of a menace. It's good to drink two and a half litres of water a day anyway, as this helps to lower the salt levels in your blood, which helps blood pressure and general health too.

Eye conditions

Most of us value our sight more than any other sense, and would fight tooth and nail to preserve it. The most common age-related eye conditions include cataracts, glaucoma and diabetic retinopathy, but one of the perhaps lesser-known conditions is age-related macular degeneration (AMD). This is a disease that gradually destroys sharp, central vision and ultimately leads to our eye or eyes struggling with fine sight details. In some cases AMD advances so slowly that we hardly notice any change in vision, but for others the disease progresses faster and may lead to a loss of vision in both eyes.

Research into what we can do to reduce the risk of AMD isn't conclusive, but there is some interesting research, which suggests that our diets can have an impact. Smoking is a major risk factor for both AMD and cataracts, and if you have the early stages of AMD your doctor will probably encourage you to quit, as you can slow down the disease quite profoundly by doing so. When we look beyond giving up smoking, it does seem that an antioxidant-rich diet with a good variety of fruit and vegetables is once more where we should focus our attention, as it's thought that the physical changes which occur in the eye are largely down to free radical damage. And as with most areas of our body, the eye doesn't just need you to be tucking into vegetables and fruits. There is some evidence to suggest that oily fish ◆ can also reduce your risk of developing AMD.

Read more on:
◆ Pages 17–18 & 95

Smoked mackerel pâté, page 217

Antioxidant nutrients found in fruit and vegetables hold some power when it comes to protecting our eyes from AMD; they like to scavenge and react with free radicals to prevent them from damaging us. Admittedly research has tended to be shown in a laboratory setting, so we don't know yet how this will translate if we eat a diet rich in these specific nutrients; but since they have been shown more widely to be great for us, let's follow this line of thought.

The key eye-benefiting antioxidant nutrients are vitamin C and the carotenoids lutein and zeaxanthin. Vitamin C is much talked about, but the highest hitters with the stranger-sounding carotenoids are spinach, kale, broccoli and red and orange peppers. Zeaxanthin is found in greatest quantities in mangoes, oranges, red and orange peppers, nectarines, papayas, squashes and honeydew melons. The good news for lutein and zeaxanthin is that unlike vitamin C, which is very sensitive to heat and time, the carotenoids are more robust and don't tend to deteriorate as rapidly with cooking. Our body's ability to absorb and use these carotenoids also improves with cooking, so small ravioli stuffed with ricotta and spinach or a thick Tuscan-style bean soup with peppers and curly kale would be a couple of delicious options to try – if the spinach was raw or just steamed you'd glean some useful vitamin C too.

However, rather than feeling as if you have to eat something rich in lutein or zeaxanthin every day, I would instead suggest that you ensure you have them as part of your five-a-day mantra and try to have a good spectrum of colours to maximise your chances of gleaning a range of antioxidants. One of my main reasons for suggesting that we shouldn't focus on eating only these specific fruits and vegetables is that to see the benefits we should be having a diet containing about 6mg of lutein daily – and this would amount to eating about 200g (3½ cups) of spinach every day, which is an awful lot. Lutein and zeaxanthin supplement tablets can be bought in health food shops, but I wouldn't recommend taking them unless recommended by a doctor or dietitian. It's very easy to take supplements that are unnecessary so you're much better off ensuring that your diet is rich in a good spectrum of vegetables and fruits, including those rich in lutein and zeaxanthin.

Dementia

As we get older we fear a deterioration in the way our brain functions perhaps even more than cancer or any other disease. Much of this fear surrounds dementia, for the simple reason that it is very ill understood and until you've had someone close to you develop this disease, nothing prepares you for the immense challenges it presents. Also, unlike cancer and heart disease, where there are public awareness campaigns the issue of dementia is still seen as something to be hidden, and admitting that there is any presence of brain disease is something very few are happy to do. Research into dementia is slow because people are far more likely to support cancer research than contribute to an Alzheimer's charity. Dementia is progressive, which means that the symptoms will gradually get worse, but how fast it progresses will largely depend on the individual and on how early on they can access support and treatments.

It can be a very difficult issue to bring up and discuss within families, so many people would prefer to try to ignore the problems; to broach the idea of someone dear to you having problems with their brain is often met with denial and aggression. It is all in all a very upsetting problem, but one that can have a big impact on our quality of life.

It's hard to cover all the elements of how food and dementia influence each other, but I have a real 'bee in my bonnet' about the fact that the concern for dementia sufferers' nutritional wellbeing doesn't feature high enough on the list of priorities in care homes, hospitals or if someone is living alone. It absolutely should be at the top of the list, because it can have such a profound effect on the disease and the lives of all concerned. Care homes can charge a significant fee so there is no excuse for poor-quality food, even on the tightest budgets. I think it's atrocious how many dementia sufferers and those who are generally old and frail have their food plonked in front of them with no one to help them eat it. Someone should be there to sit and take the stalks off grapes, peel a clementine, cajole without pestering someone who has a poor appetite, help them to eat and ensure that if they don't manage to eat much during that meal this is noted and monitored.

Dementia is seldom the same for everyone, but we usually experience memory loss, a change in moods, anxiety, depression and aggression. It can be a very disempowering condition, and is often frightening as we don't understand what's happening to us. Part of the problem, too, is that dementia can really start to affect our ability to communicate, which can lead to isolation and our needs won't always be met. As you might expect, our ability to carry out even the most basic of everyday tasks gradually disappears and we become more and more reliant on others.

Diverticular disease

Chicken &
chickpea
burgers,
page 212

As we get older our gut changes in all sorts of ways, even when our diet apparently stays the same. We have some ideas as to why this happens although it's usually a combination of things – being less active, certain drugs and our gut 'holding' upset and tension inside. This can be a sensitive subject, as we may look all right on the outside, but tension, grief or upset of any sort can make bowel movements difficult. Sometimes the less we're able to go to the toilet the more uptight we get, making our gut even more unpredictable. All in all, the more we can do to try to reduce the anxiety surrounding our bowel habits, by doing gentle exercises, eating nourishing good-for-the-gut foods, drinking plenty of water, and trying to reduce stress and boost happy endorphin levels, the sooner our gut will settle down. Do check out one of my favourite anti-anxiety machines, the Pzizz machine, as this meditation device can make a real difference to the way the gut behaves.

Being constipated is one of the things that can increase the risk of developing diverticular disease, which is thought to be present in at least half of the population over 65. Diverticular disease happens when the walls of the intestine weaken, forming pockets or sacs (diverticula). Many people never know they have diverticula in their intestine because they have no symptoms, and luckily only 25 per cent of sufferers are struck down with symptoms of severe abdominal pain, intermittent diarrhoea and constipation.

Diverticula often develop because our diet is relatively deficient in fibre-rich foods, which help to prevent constipation – it's the straining involved in passing a stool that weakens the intestinal walls, causing diverticula to form. So preventing constipation is important to ensure that diverticula don't develop in the first place.

Sometimes diverticula can become infected and cause rectal bleeding, pain and fever; if untreated this can prove to be serious, as the infection can become widespread and cause all sorts of complications. If you're diagnosed with an infection, the advice completely changes – the last thing you need is roughage, as it's too much for a sore, infected intestine to deal with. You need a low-fibre diet, which means switching from high-fibre foods to white rice, pasta, white fish such as grilled Dover sole, seabass and some fresh prawns, chicken, a few cooked (not raw) fruits and vegetables. For the immediate future, stay away from vegetables and fruits with seeds such as tomatoes, courgettes, marrows, grapes (this is simply because sometimes seeds get trapped in the diverticula, aggravating the infection), and wind-inducing vegetables like Brussels sprouts, cabbages, beans and lentils.

Read
more on:
◆ Pages
104–105

Vegetable soup
with lime
& herbs,
page 230

Once the infection has been treated successfully (which most likely will need antibiotics, as a gut infection is a serious medical condition), look to see if you can improve your gut bacterial flora. First take a combined prebiotic and probiotic supplement ◆ , to help ensure that the bacterial balance in your gut returns to normal after the course of antibiotics. Then, once your infection has cleared up, start gently building up your fibre intake, so that your gut returns to a good non-constipated state. But gently does it.

Recovering from surgery

We are at our most vulnerable when we've undergone an operation, because the operation puts our body under a lot of strain – the physical trauma of being cut into and the hormonal responses to being operated on can use up a lot of stores, such as fat, muscle, vitamins and minerals. Even with the best hygiene standards in the operating theatre, any operation introduces bacteria and viruses into our body that can challenge our immune system. Furthermore, if we're undergoing surgery it's possible that we've not been feeling at our best for a while, may not have been eating well and may have other health problems that will hinder our recovery. It's unusual that we go into the operating theatre feeling 100 per cent. And indeed, after the operation it's highly likely that we'll have a few days when our body is unable to tolerate much, if any, food, as the anaesthetic often affects the bowel.

Even for people who are in theory able to cope with a nourishing meal, hospitals and care homes can be atrocious at providing appetising, nutritious foods and ensuring that patients eat enough of it to enable their bodies to recover. So often it is down to us, the relatives, to take the issue of eating for recovery into our own hands. Being able to look after someone we care about in this way can be incredibly valuable, as we so often feel helpless.

I want to take you through the foods and nutrients needed to recover that are often contrary to those that patients and relatives think they need. It's not all about fruits and vegetables rich in the skin- and body-repairing nutrients such as vitamin C. Of course vitamin C is a valuable nutrient but when our body is recovering from surgery or any situation that has depleted our energy stores, we need more than anything to eat plenty of calories. Our body needs a plentiful supply of calories to repair skin and muscle, build new bone, fight other infections, and prevent any further loss of the padding we have underneath our skin. But often there is another challenge, that of not having much of an appetite, so we need to focus on small amounts of nourishing, calorie-rich foods. This is not the moment for nibbling on a few grapes thinking they're a good source of vitamin C – your body needs fat, carbohydrate and protein. In particular, being ill or having an operation often depletes your protein reserves, and although this is putting somewhat complex physiological processes into very simple terms, each meal you eat should include a protein-rich food as well as a good source of starchy carbohydrate with some good fat alongside it.

Fine-tuning the fibre

When recovering from an operation, you may find that high-fibre, carbohydrate-rich foods fill you up too quickly. A good alternative is a white bread sandwich with a protein-rich filling such as ham (wafer-thin honey roast ham, proscuitto etc.), fish such as smoked trout or mackerel, eggs (ensuring they're hard-boiled to prevent salmonella poisoning), chicken or cheese. You may find a big steak off-putting, but a small portion of shepherd's pie, made with beef or lamb mince in a rich gravy and topped with a crunchy layer of buttery mashed potato, could hit the spot.

However, a common side-effect of surgery or being bedridden for a while is constipation, and if you start eating white bread and pasta instead of the wholemeal variety you may not get enough fibre to kick-start and encourage the bowel to get moving. One way round this would be to eat fruit and vegetable options such as compote of fruits, poached fruit with custard or panacotta, juices, soups or porridge with honey and berries on top. In order to ensure that the meal isn't full of too much fibre and not enough calories, the solution would be to add something high in fat or sugar to up its energy content: stirring cream into soups; adding honey or brown sugar to porridge; using thick Greek-style yoghurt and full cream milk on cereals.

Small, nutritionally powerful and delicious

Recovering from any illness, especially if you've had an operation or have pressure sores, requires a plentiful supply of vitamin C and other skin- and tissue-healing nutrients such as zinc (see below). Stir thick yoghurt into a home-made smoothie, serve cream with strawberries, bake peaches with dark muscovado-style sugar or maple syrup, or have a vegetable or fruit juice in between meals. Make sure it's not too close to a mealtime, as liquid fills you up so quickly that to have a juice as a starter or a soup could just scupper the chance of being able to eat anything more substantial. Whereas I don't usually like nouvelle cuisine, preferring to cook big pots of something hearty in the middle of the table that everyone dips into, this is an instance where a little espresso cup of a creamy leek and potato soup mid-meal could just be what's needed – small and delicately presented, it will often be just what you fancy too.

Lack of zinc can exacerbate any poor appetite – the less zinc-rich foods we eat, the less inclined we are to want to eat; it's a vicious cycle we would do good to break. Zinc-rich foods include lean red meat, nuts, seeds, shellfish such as oysters and prawns, crumbly cheese such as Cheshire, Lancashire and Parmesan, and wholegrains, but while I'm not usually a fan of unnecessary vitamin and mineral supplements it may be a good idea, especially if you're off your food, to take a 200–220mg zinc sulphate supplement two or three times a day (discuss it with your doctor to ensure that this complements any other drugs, as sometimes they can interfere). This may not only bring back the appetite but also helps with wound healing, etc.

Bolognese sauce, page 210

Low iron levels can be common after an operation (when you will have lost some blood), and also if you've not been eating well for a while. Check your iron level, which is linked to your haemoglobin level, as low haemoglobin levels not only hinder healing but can also make us exhausted and have low moods. Even if our haemoglobin level is normal our ferritin (iron store) levels can be low, which can lead to hair loss and poor wound healing, so you may also like to check this out with your doctor. As with zinc, if your appetite is off it may be that an iron supplement providing something like 200mg of ferrous sulphate (iron) may e useful, although some people don't tolerate this well. It can cause constipation or diarrhoea, in which case discuss with your doctor whether one of the more gentle iron supplements might be suitable alongside focusing on this aspect of your diet.

Vitamin D is vital for wound healing, and since our ability to synthesise this vitamin in our skin decreases with age and can be particularly poor if you're spending a lot of time indoors recuperating, it's even more important to take a 10mcg (400 IU) supplement each day.

Drinking enough

It can be tempting to think that taking lots of mineral and vitamin supplements will get you better more quickly, but this isn't the case – there is nothing better, nothing more nourishing in its truest and most complete sense, than eating and drinking well. You need to keep up your fluid intake and usually I would suggest keeping the majority of the fluid as water, as there is nothing more hydrating. When you're trying to increase your calorie, protein, fat and other nutrient intakes it can be good to include milky drinks, which provide protein, fat, calories, calcium, zinc – the full-fat versions are the most nutrient-dense and you can add honey to them. It may surprise you to hear that I'm also a fan of cordials, squashes and juices, as they provide some glucose, which can be a good source of energy. Or indeed, a cup of tea can be milky sweet and makes the perfect boost with a biscuit ◆ while soups make a nourishing drink too.

Read more on:
◆ *Pages 33–36*

Tooth decay

We become far more susceptible to tooth decay as we get older, and of course losing our teeth and having to rely on dentures, is not as valuable as having your own set of healthy teeth. One of the biggest problems for older people who have been unwell for a while is that their dentures can become less well-fitting, as the gums can retract and become sore if the body is run down – all of this can put you off your food, and here starts another destructive vicious cycle.

Some medications, like antibiotics and laxatives, can be very high in sugar, while others can exacerbate a more common ageing scenario: the decrease in the amount of saliva we produce. All these factors have a negative impact on our teeth, so the more we can do to prevent tooth decay when we're older the better. I bring up this subject now because I've mentioned above that sweet drinks can be a good way, as can biscuits, etc., to boost your calorie intake when you're recovering from an illness or operation, but too much sweet stuff, even if it's just a seemingly harmless cup of sweet tea, can ultimately cause tooth decay. So just watch that you're not having too much and on a too frequent a basis – five sweet hits during a day is about the right sort of level, as this gives the mouth enough time in between to recover and rebalance its acidity levels (which go up when you've eaten something sweet). This highlights a real problem with relying on some of the very thick and sweet supplement drinks – using a straw can help reduce the impact on the teeth.

It can also give us an added impetus to think of savoury alternatives to sweet treats, especially if you think you're treating by giving them another slice of cake when perhaps a sandwich or a slice of toast with some cheese on top would actually be far more nourishing snack and better for their teeth.

Good oral hygiene and using a fluoride-rich toothpaste can help too – most pastes contain fluoride, it's true, but you can get some especially high-fluoride ones for older people who are most at risk of tooth decay (wait 30 minutes after eating before you brush too).

Dementia care

The foods we eat can have a very significant influence our lives, and not only on our physical health. The level to which we're well nourished can have an impact on our moods, and when it comes to reducing the risk or the progression of dementia, although research is still in its infancy, there are a few very important relationships between nutrients and brain health that are worth exploring.

The first of these surrounds the overall levels of nourishment and the likelihood of developing dementia. We do know that having a nourishing, well-rounded diet gives our brain the best chance of not succumbing to the disease, because strong relationships exist between eating well and reducing the likelihood of suffering from a stroke, for instance; but over and above eating a well-balanced diet, full of wholegrain, fruits and vegetables, there is some new research that suggests that the omega-3 fatty acids ◆ in particular can play a significant role in reducing some of the risk. Also, when dementia is diagnosed, it looks as if eating a diet rich in omega-3 fatty acids could help to slow down the progression of the disease. It's all well and good saying that we should therefore be eating a couple of portions of oily fish a week, but the other far greater challenge we face with dementia is that as the disease progresses, our ability and desire to eat deteriorates. Which is really why we need to focus on what we can do to meet these practical challenges head on.

Read more on:
◆ Pages 17–18 & 95

My mum's chicken pie, page 211

There are some very practical issues that dementia presents, not least the fact that memory loss and confusion mean that some people may forget to eat; from one meal to another, time of day and the importance of eating can be lost and when dementia hits hard, even the presence of food on a plate in front of you doesn't necessarily mean you'll know it's there to be eaten. Our ability to judge temperature can disappear too, so if food is served too hot it can burn our lips or throat, and physical skills like keeping our mouths closed while food is inside, to help us chew and swallow, can become difficult.

We may not be able or be safe enough to cook or prepare food on our own, while depression, low energy and constipation can all make eating difficult. Unlike when we have food battles with our young children, when we're dealing with an adult, particularly our parents, who is strong and possesses the language to lash out, much as we try not to let words and actions wound us, they do – we're all human and have our limits. It sounds so basic, and I don't mean it to be patronising, but there are a few things to try to keep in the forefront of your mind, or to write down and stick on the wall as visual mantras.

Try to keep calm

A calm, regular routine is reassuring for someone with dementia – even being ten minutes out in a routine, or sitting at a different table, or with friends they don't usually eat with, can upset them. The requirement to always stick to the same routine can be isolating for you, the carer, as your whole day is dictated by something that used to be flexible and sociable. One way around this is to feed them in the same way, at the same time, and then for you yourself to eat with friends afterwards. You will then be more able to enjoy a nourishing meal, which is obviously very important. If we don't manage to feed ourselves properly when we're having such demands placed on us we're not going to be any use to anyone.

Try to keep things simple

While we try to juggle so many tasks when caring for someone, it can be tempting to try to hurry, which only increases the likelihood of upset and for very little food to get eaten. Because concentration needs to be maximised to enable the person we're caring for to eat and focus on swallowing or getting the food from fork to mouth, etc., it helps not to have the radio or the TV on as a rule. This said, I do have some patients who find that listening to meditative music can help take some of the aggression out of the situation if the meal's heading that way. It can certainly help us to step back for a minute and find the strength we need to go back with a calm attitude.

If you're finding that the person you're looking after is frustrated by not being able to eat when the sole focus is on eating, you might find that sitting in front of the TV with a plate of something easy to nibble, such as sandwiches or crisps, or soft fruits such as bananas, could just mean that these get eaten while they're being distracted by the programme. One thing to remember is that if they're very upset or agitated, or if they're drowsy and not very responsive, feeding can cause choking – so try to leave a bit of time before you try, and seek advice and help if you're having problems with these aspects.

As the dementia progresses it's highly likely that appetite and ability to eat will change – this can sometimes be sudden, though it's more common for it to fall off more subtly – so you will probably have to become flexible in your routine. Don't feel that changes in appetite or ability to eat are always down to the disease itself – sometimes medication can put them off their food and interfere with hunger messages in the brain. We also shouldn't forget the simple fact that sometimes they can't remember if they've eaten, so

Chicken with winter vegetables, page 214

they may say they want more food when physically they don't need it.

I think we tend to assume that as dementia progresses the biggest challenges are weight loss, and getting them to eat enough of the right foods, but before taking you through some ideas as to how to best get around this, I want to point out that sometimes gaining too much weight becomes an issue – people with dementia can forget that they've eaten, and have difficulties knowing when to stop, as they lose the ability to register and respond to the fullness feeling. If they become overweight it not only creates physical challenges of helping them walk, etc., but poses a health risk too. So much as an occasional treat is good, keeping to the basic structure of an overall nourishing diet is best.

What to do about poor appetite

Our appetite and desire to eat anything is influenced by many factors. For instance, if we are constipated the body can take away our appetite if the gut isn't able to get rid of what it doesn't need. But many other physical problems can have an influence too, such as a sore mouth, badly fitted dentures, or just the sheer effort involved in eating for those who suffer from dementia. When our mood is low or we're angry, eating can be the last thing we feel like doing. Some of us don't like to eat on our own, which can be a real issue if we live alone or away from family.

What we do know about a poor appetite is that the less we eat, often the less we fancy eating. Malnutrition can kick in, and all sorts of problems start occurring – pressure sores, poor wound healing, depression, etc. – which would never have arisen had the person been well nourished. So if you suspect that your relative or friend in a care home isn't getting the right types of foods or that they're not getting any help with eating, make a nuisance of yourself and either try to persuade someone to sit with them while they're eating, or ask if you can bring in some food. Ensuring someone is well nourished reduces the likelihood of other medical problems arising that will require more acute and often expensive care.

If you're looking after someone at home and their appetite is off, I suggest you first try tempting their appetite. Although your individual situation will mean that some things work better than others, it will give you some ideas about how to make food as nourishing as possible, in small and practically workable ways. If you're struggling with the physical aspect of cutlery, plates, etc., seek advice and support from organisations that work with the elderly and their carers, or your doctor and district health care teams, as there are some fantastic adaptations of these home basics that can make feeding and eating far easier. Don't suffer in silence – the help is out there.

Roast mackerel with potatoes & thyme, page 215

Recipes

If I'd had room I would like to have included more recipes, but the ones in this chapter are some of my favourite staples, which you can use as a starting point. You can give them a twist – try varying the base of a soup or the topping on a pizza, for example. By changing the texture, or adding something like a dollop or two of Greek-style yoghurt and some toasted wholemeal croutons, you can make a soup you are enjoying with your young family equally appropriate for an elderly parent, spouse or friend.

I've included some recipes that use ready-made ingredients you can keep in the freezer, for times when you need to rustle up a quick but nutritious meal. While there are weekend moments that lend themselves to making your own puff pastry, you can also now buy really great ready-made pastries that don't contain the hydrogenated fats we've worried about in the past. Rolled out and filled with fruits, they make a delicious contribution towards your five-a-day target.

Recipe index

Chickpea, tomato & sausage hot pot

SERVES 4

2 tbsp olive oil

2 large onions, roughly chopped

4 cloves garlic, thinly sliced

1 leek, finely chopped

400g (14oz) good quality, lean sausages (I like to use a variety)

1 tbsp dried chilli flakes (red pepper flakes)

175ml (¾ cup) dry sherry, or white or red wine

8 ripe tomatoes, roughly chopped

200g (1½ cups) canned chickpeas, drained and rinsed

1 bay leaf

1 small bunch of fresh parsley, roughly chopped

Warm the olive oil in a deep, heavy-based pan or flameproof casserole dish. Add the onions and cook over a medium heat for a few minutes. Add the garlic and leek, and cook with the onions until they turn a pale golden colour.

Cut each sausage into four and add them to the onion pot along with the dried chilli flakes. Pour in the sherry or wine, bring to the boil and add the tomatoes, chickpeas and bay leaf. Bring to the boil, then turn down to a simmer and leave to cook, half-covered, for 45 minutes.

Stir from time to time and, if necessary, add a little water to make a thick, rich tomato sauce. Just before serving, stir in the parsley.

Other herbs work well, such as chopped coriander (cilantro) or torn basil.

This is also delicious served with little dumplings or mashed potato, or it can be blended to make a scrumptious soup.

Pearled spelt, goat's cheese & chard risotto

SERVES 4

250g (9oz) pearled spelt
½ tbsp olive or rapeseed oil
2 medium shallots or 1 small onion, finely chopped
1 litre (4 cups) hot vegetable stock
2 handfuls of chard or spinach leaves
50g (2oz) soft goat's cheese
freshly grated Parmesan or Pecorino cheese
salt and ground black pepper

Soak the spelt in cold water for 10 minutes. Heat the oil in a large pan and cook the shallots until soft but not brown. Drain the spelt, add it to the shallots and pour in one-third of the stock. Bring to the boil then turn the heat down to a simmer and gradually add the remaining stock a ladleful at a time, stirring constantly.

When the spelt is cooked but not mushy (as you still want it to have a slight bite to it), tear the chard leaves, stir them in and leave them to soften for 1–2 minutes. Add the cheese and season to taste.

This risotto can be made with Arborio rice instead of spelt and all kinds of other ingredients, such as mushrooms, peas or broad beans (fava beans), which can be thrown in from frozen at the chard stage, as they only take a couple of minutes to cook.

Butternut squash & red lentil dahl

SERVES 3–4

1 medium squash, unpeeled and
   halved
300g (1⅔ cups) red lentils, rinsed
1 tsp ground cumin
½ tsp ground turmeric
1 cinnamon stick
2cm (¾ in) piece of fresh root ginger,
   peeled and grated
1 litre (4 cups) hot water
rice, chapattis or naan bread, to serve

FOR THE TARKA

1 tbsp olive oil
2 red onions, thinly sliced
2 garlic cloves, thinly sliced
1 red large chilli, cut into thin strips

Preheat the oven to 190°C/375°F (170°C fan oven) mark 5. Place the squash on a baking sheet and bake for 30–40 minutes until it turns golden and soft. Allow to cool slightly and then discard the seeds, scoop out the flesh and set aside.

Meanwhile, put the lentils, cumin, turmeric, cinnamon, ginger and hot water into a pan. Bring to the boil, then simmer over a low heat, stirring occasionally, for 30 minutes or until very soft.

Remove the cinnamon stick from the lentils and discard. Add the squash, stirring to break up any lumps.

To make the tarka, heat the olive oil in a frying pan, add the onions and cook on a very low heat until golden and caramelised. Add the garlic and chilli to the tarka and cook over a low heat for 10 minutes. Serve the dahl in bowls with a spoonful of the tarka to garnish.

Beans with tomato, coriander & coconut milk

SERVES 4–6

400g (2¼ cups) dried haricot beans or
    chickpeas, soaked overnight
1 tbsp olive oil
2 medium onions, thinly sliced
3 garlic cloves, finely chopped
seeds from 8 green cardamoms
2 tsp coriander seeds
1 tsp yellow mustard seeds
1 tsp cumin seeds
2 tsp ground turmeric
salt and ground black pepper
3 small hot chillies, deseeded and
    finely chopped
2 x 400g (14oz) cans chopped
    plum tomatoes
400ml (1¾ cups) water
a pinch of sugar
250ml (1 cup) coconut milk
a large handful of fresh coriander
    leaves
juice of 2 limes or lemons

Rinse the beans and cook in fresh water for 1 hour or until tender. Heat the oil in a large, deep pan, add the onions and cook over a medium heat until softened and slightly golden. Add the garlic and cook for 2–3 minutes.

Crush the cardamom, coriander and mustard seeds using a pestle and mortar or heavy rolling pin, then stir them into the onions. Add the cumin seeds, ground turmeric and salt and pepper, and cook for 5 minutes.

Add the chillies, tomatoes, water, sugar and cooked beans. Simmer over a low heat for 35–40 minutes. Stir the coconut milk into the sauce, simmer for 5 minutes, then add the coriander leaves (cilantro) and the lime juice.

Alternatively, you can use 3 × 400g (14oz) cans beans or chickpeas, drained and rinsed.

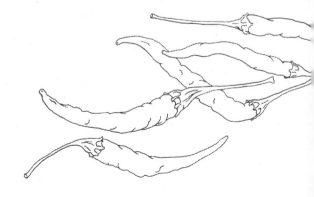

Pearled spelt with broad beans, asparagus & dill

SERVES **4**

125g (2 cups) fresh spinach, washed
50g (heaped ⅓ cup) broad beans (fava beans),
    blanched for 1 minute
50g (⅓ cup) peas, thawed if frozen, blanched for 1 minute
8 asparagus spears, blanched for 2 minutes
225g (8oz) pearled spelt, cooked for 20 minutes
a handful of fresh dill, torn into small fronds
4 tbsp extra virgin olive oil
juice of 1 lime or lemon
1 tsp finely chopped chilli (optional)
salt and ground black pepper

Put the spinach in a dry pan over a low heat and cook in the water that clings to the leaves after washing for 3 minutes or until wilted. Remove quickly and drain in a colander.

Put the broad beans in a bowl and mix with the peas, asparagus, pearled spelt and spinach. Add the dill and dress with olive oil, lime juice and chilli, if using. Season and toss together lightly with your fingers. Serve quickly while the flavours are fresh.

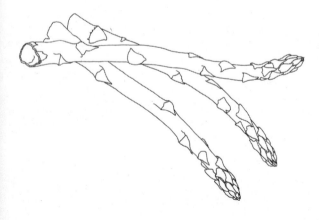

Cauliflower cheese

SERVES 4

25g (1¾ tbsp) butter, plus extra for greasing
1 large white cauliflower and 1 large green cauliflower,
   trimmed and broken into florets
25g (3 tbsp) plain (all-purpose) flour
600ml (1 pint) milk
100g (1 cup) mature Cheddar cheese, grated
1 tbsp Dijon mustard, or 1 tsp made-up English mustard
a pinch of grated nutmeg
ground black pepper
25g (½ cup) fresh wholemeal breadcrumbs
50g (¾ cup) freshly grated Parmesan cheese

Preheat the oven to 200°C/400°F (180°C fan oven) mark 6. Lightly grease an ovenproof dish that is large enough to hold the cauliflower in one layer. Steam or boil the cauliflower for 5–6 minutes until just tender, then drain and set aside.

Melt the butter in a pan over a low heat. Add the flour and stir for 1 minute, without browning. Remove from the heat and gradually beat in the milk. Return the pan to the heat and simmer gently, stirring frequently, for 10 minutes or until the sauce is thickened and creamy.

Remove the pan from the heat and stir in three quarters of the Cheddar cheese and the mustard. Season with nutmeg and pepper. Put the cauliflower in the greased dish and pour the sauce over it.

Mix together the breadcrumbs, Parmesan and the remaining Cheddar cheese, and sprinkle evenly over the cauliflower and sauce. Bake for 25–30 minutes until browned and bubbling. Serve immediately.

If using non-dairy milk, butter and cheese, you might want to add other vegetables, such as sautéed mushrooms and herbs, to the sauce to give it some extra flavour.

Bolognese sauce

SERVES 8

3 tbsp olive oil

50g (2oz) smoked streaky bacon, cut into small pieces

1 onion, finely chopped

2 celery sticks, finely chopped

2 carrots, finely chopped

2 garlic cloves, finely chopped

1 tsp fresh thyme leaves

1 bay leaf

1 tsp dried oregano

400g (14oz) can chopped tomatoes

1 tbsp tomato purée (paste)

1 tsp anchovy essence or anchovy sauce

1 tbsp Worcestershire sauce

900g (2lb) good quality lean minced (ground) beef

125g (½ cup) fresh chicken livers, finely chopped (optional)

750ml (3¼ cups) dry red wine or water

1 litre (4 cups) hot chicken, beef or lamb stock

salt and ground black pepper

Heat 1 tbsp oil in a large, heavy-based pan and fry the bacon until crispy. Add the onion, celery, carrots, garlic, thyme, bay leaf and oregano, and cook over a medium heat until the vegetables have softened. Stir in the tomatoes, tomato purée, anchovy essence and Worcestershire sauce.

In a separate frying pan, heat 1 tbsp of oil and fry the minced beef in small batches until browned. Drain off any fat and add to the tomato mixture. Add another 1 tbsp oil to the pan and fry the chicken livers, if using, until brown and crusty, then add to the tomato and mince mixture. Deglaze the frying pan with 2–3 tbsp red wine, scraping any sediment from the bottom. Pour the remaining wine and the stock into the tomato and meat mixture. Bring to the boil, reduce the heat and simmer, stirring occasionally, for 2 hours, adding a little water if it gets too dry. Season to taste.

My mum's chicken pie

SERVES 3–4

    butter, for greasing
    2 medium onions, roughly chopped
    1 garlic clove, peeled
    500g (1lb 2oz) cooked chicken meat, breast and legs
    juice of 1 lemon
    a few leaves of fresh sage or a few sprigs of parsley
    ground black pepper
    375g (13oz) shortcrust pastry (pie dough), thawed if frozen
    1 egg, beaten

Preheat the oven to 200°C/400°F (180°C fan oven) gas 6. Grease a
25.5cm (10in) pie dish. Put the onions, garlic, chicken, lemon juice, fresh
herbs and pepper into a food processor or mincer (grinder) and mince until
you have a mixture that resembles chunky sausage meat.

Roll out half the pastry and line the pie dish. Put in the chicken mixture and
spread it level. Roll out the remaining pastry and put it on top. Squeeze
the edges together. Cut a couple of slits in the middle of the pie to allow
steam to escape while it's cooking. Brush the pie with the egg, and bake
for 50 minutes–1 hour until the pastry is golden brown.

*If you make your own pastry you could use half white and half
wholemeal (wholewheat) flour.*

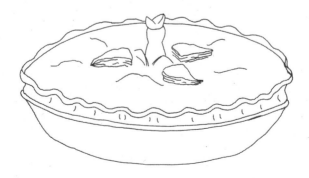

Chicken & chickpea burgers

SERVES 4

450g (1lb) roasted chicken
200g (1½ cups) canned chickpeas, drained and rinsed
1 small onion, roughly chopped
1 garlic clove, roughly chopped
2 tsp finely chopped fresh sage
175g (3 cups) wholemeal (wholewheat) breadcrumbs
1 egg, beaten
salt and ground black pepper

Put the chicken, chickpeas, onion and garlic in a food processor or mincer (grinder) and mince to combine. Alternatively, chop finely and mash together with a fork, or put the ingredients in a clean plastic bag, tie the end, then put on a hard surface and hit with a rolling pin until mashed together.

Put the mixture in a bowl, add the sage, one third of the breadcrumbs and enough of the egg to bind the mixture without it becoming too sloppy. Season to taste.

Spread the remaining breadcrumbs on a large baking sheet and, taking a handful of mixture at a time, form a ball, then roll in the breadcrumbs until completely coated. Grill until the coating turns golden brown. Serve immediately.

Try replacing the chickpeas with broad beans (fava beans) or canned beans such as haricot, butter (lima) or borlotti (cranberry beans). The burgers can also be made with other roasted meats such as ham, roast pork or beef.

Tandoori chicken

SERVES 4

1.25kg (2¾lb) chicken pieces, legs and/or breasts, skinned
3 tbsp lemon juice
450ml (2 cups) Greek yogurt
1 onion, coarsely chopped
1 garlic clove, chopped
2.5cm (1in) piece fresh root ginger, peeled and chopped
1–2 hot green chillies, roughly sliced
2 tsp garam masala
coarse sea salt
lime or lemon wedges, to serve

Cut each chicken leg into two pieces and each breast into four. Make two deep slits crossways on the meaty parts, making sure that they don't start at an edge and that they are deep enough to reach the bone. Spread the chicken pieces out on two large platters. Sprinkle one side with a pinch of salt and half the lemon juice, and rub in. Turn the pieces over and repeat on the second side. Set aside for 20 minutes.

Put the yogurt, onion, garlic, ginger, chillies and garam masala in a blender or food processor and whiz until smooth. Place in a bowl along with the chicken. Rub the marinade into the slits in the meat, then cover and chill for 1–2 hours, or overnight if possible.

When you're ready to cook, preheat the oven to 240°C/475°F (220°C fan oven) mark 9 and set a shelf in the top third of the oven where it is hottest. Put the chicken in a single layer on a large, shallow baking tray and bake for 20–25 minutes until cooked through. Lift the chicken pieces out of their juices and serve with lime or lemon wedges.

Chicken with winter vegetables

SERVES 4

1 medium-sized chicken, giblets removed
large bunch of flat-leafed parsley
4 bunches of thyme
3 bay leaves
1 small head each of fennel and celeriac, finely chopped
1 leek, roughly chopped
4 carrots, chopped into large pieces
750ml bottle dry white wine
450g (1lb) small waxy (boiling) potatoes, peeled
salt and ground black pepper
Dijon mustard, to serve

Preheat the oven to 200°C/400°F (180°C fan oven) mark 6. Put the chicken in a large, heavy casserole dish. Remove the leaves from the parsley and set them aside. Put the parsley stalks, thyme, bay leaves, fennel, celeriac, leek and carrots into the casserole dish. Pour in the wine, season with salt and pepper and cover with a lid. Cook in the oven for 2½ hours.

Remove and discard the parsley stalks and thyme stems. Transfer the chicken to a serving platter and cover it with clingfilm (plastic wrap). Put the potatoes in a pan of lightly salted cold water, bring to the boil and simmer until cooked. Finely chop the reserved parsley leaves and add them to the cooked vegetables, check the seasoning and stir well.

Serve the thick parsley and vegetable soup as a first course, then serve the chicken and potatoes with the mustard.

Roast mackerel with potatoes & thyme

SERVES 2

300g (2 cups) small new potatoes, cut into 2cm (¾in) slices
3 tbsp olive oil
4 tbsp fresh thyme leaves
salt and ground black pepper
1 tbsp sherry vinegar
2 large or 3–4 small mackerel fillets, cleaned and deboned
watercress and tomato salad, to serve

Preheat the oven to 180°C/350°F (160°C fan oven) mark 4. Put the potatoes into a shallow dish, drizzle with 1 tbsp oil and sprinkle with 3 tbsp thyme leaves, salt and lots of pepper. Coat the potatoes well, then bake in the oven for 40 minutes or until golden and tender when pricked with a fork.

Mix the remaining oil, the sherry vinegar and the remaining thyme with salt and pepper in a small bowl. Put the mackerel skin-side up on top of the potatoes and spoon the herby dressing over them. Put it back into the oven and cook for 15–20 minutes until the mackerel is cooked and slightly crispy. Serve with a watercress and tomato salad.

This recipe works equally well for any oily fish, such as herrings and sardines, although the cooking time will change depending on the size of the fish.

Spicy fish casserole

SERVES 4

400g (14oz) new potatoes, scrubbed and cut into thick slices
3 tomatoes, peeled and quartered
3 garlic cloves, chopped
2.5cm (1in) piece of fresh green
    or red chilli, finely chopped,
½ tsp paprika
½ tsp ground cumin
juice of 1 lemon
500g (1lb 2oz) white fish fillets, skinned
25g (1 cup) fresh flat-leafed parsley, chopped
2 fresh mint sprigs, leaves chopped
4 large handfuls of spinach
ground black pepper

Put the potatoes, tomatoes, garlic, chilli, paprika and cumin into a large pan and add 1 litre (4 cups) water and half the lemon juice. Simmer for 25 minutes or until the potatoes are tender.

Add the fish fillets and cook for another 10 minutes, then gently break up the fish into smaller pieces and add the herbs and the spinach. Cook for a further 1 minute, then stir. Season with pepper and add the remaining lemon juice.

*The flavours of this dish will develop if
you cover it well and chill it, then eat the following day.*

Smoked mackerel pâté

SERVES 4 AS A STARTER

    200g (7oz) smoked mackerel fillets (without pepper), skins removed
    200g (7oz) ricotta cheese
    a squeeze of fresh lemon juice
    2 tbsp Greek yogurt
    ground black pepper

Add all the ingredients to a food processor or blender, season with ground black pepper and whiz together until smooth.

Spread the pâté on toast or flatbreads or use in sandwiches. For sandwich rolls, spread over fresh, soft, good-quality white or wholemeal (wholewheat) bread, crusts removed, then roll up. Cut across the roll into slices.

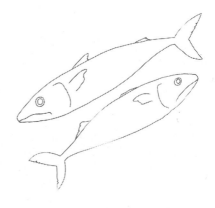

Roasted tomato & couscous salad

SERVES 6–8

16 large ripe plum or round tomatoes

2 tbsp muscovado or soft brown sugar

4 tbsp olive oil, plus extra for drizzling

2 tbsp balsamic vinegar

coarse sea salt and black pepper

2 onions, thinly sliced

250g (1 ¼ cups) brown rice, mograbiah, pearled spelt or quinoa

400ml (1 ¾ cups) chicken or vegetable stock

a pinch of saffron threads

250g (1 ½ cups) couscous

1 tbsp chopped fresh tarragon

1 tbsp nigella seeds

1 tsp finely chopped sun-dried tomatoes

100g (½ cup) of labneh or thick yogurt

a handful of stoned (pitted) green olives, sliced

Preheat the oven to 150°C/300°F (130°C fan oven) mark 2. Cut the tomatoes into quarters lengthways, or slice them in half if using round tomatoes, and put on a baking tray, skin-side down. Sprinkle with sugar, 2 tbsp olive oil, the balsamic vinegar and salt and pepper. Roast in the oven for 2 hours or until the tomatoes have lost most of their moisture.

Put the remaining olive oil in a large pan and sauté the onions over a high heat for 10–12 minutes, stirring occasionally, until a dark golden colour. Put the rice into a large pan of slightly salted boiling water and simmer for 15 minutes or until tender but not mushy. Drain and rinse under cold water.

Boil the stock in a pan. Add the saffron and a little salt. Put the couscous in a large bowl and pour the boiling stock over it. Cover and leave for 10 minutes. Fluff up with a fork. Add the rice, tomatoes and juices, onions and oils, tarragon, half the nigella seeds and the sun-dried tomatoes. Adjust the seasoning. Serve at room temperature with a good spoonful of labneh and a drizzle of oil, the remaining nigella seeds and the sliced olives.

Tomato &
herb salad

SERVES 4

    a handful each of basil, mint
        (spearmint – *Mentha spicata* – is best for salad if you can find it),
        curly-leafed parsley and chives
    3 handfuls each of Italian rocket (arugula) and ruby chard
    4–6 ripe baby tomatoes, quartered
    1 ripe avocado, peeled and sliced
    extra virgin olive oil, for drizzling
    leaves from 1 thyme sprig

Tear the basil, finely chop the mint, parsley and chives, and put into a salad bowl. Throw in the rocket and chard leaves, the tomatoes and the avocado. Drizzle with enough olive oil to lightly coat the leaves, scatter with the thyme leaves and mix well.

Quick
Caesar salad

SERVES 2

1 slice wholemeal (wholewheat),
  white or granary bread, cubed
1 tbsp mayonnaise
1 tbsp Greek yogurt
2 garlic cloves, crushed
4 tbsp freshly grated Parmesan cheese
6 anchovy fillets, chopped
2 hard-boiled eggs, chopped
4 large handfuls of chopped cos (romaine) lettuce
ground black pepper

Preheat the oven to 230°C/450°F (210°C fan oven) mark 8. Put the bread on to a baking sheet and bake, turning twice, for 10 minutes or until golden brown all over. Allow to cool while you make the salad.

Put the mayonnaise and yogurt into a small bowl and mix in enough water to make a pourable consistency. Add the garlic, Parmesan cheese and plenty of pepper.

Put the remaining ingredients into a large salad bowl, drizzle with the creamy dressing and top with the croutons.

Serve with lean roast meats such as chicken, ham, roast beef or cold salmon, tuna, roasted cod or sea bass. It's also delicious with a simple tomato salad or some steamed asparagus or green beans.

Bought croutons can be used if you prefer.

Wild rice salad

SERVES **4**

250g (scant 1⅔ cups) wild rice
65g (½ cup) shelled pistachio nuts
150g (1 cup) soft, dried unsulphured apricots,
    soaked in hot water for 5 minutes
leaves from 1 small bunch of fresh mint
1 small bunch of rocket (arugula)
3 spring onions (scallions), roughly chopped
zest and juice of 1 lemon
2 tbsp olive oil
1 large garlic clove, crushed
sea salt and ground black pepper

Put the rice in a large pan and cover with water, bring to the boil then reduce
the heat and cook for 30–40 minutes, or until *al dente*. Drain and rinse under
cold water.

While the rice is cooking, toast the pistachio nuts in a dry pan over a
medium heat for 8–10 minutes, then coarsely chop.

Drain the apricots and chop them coarsely. In a bowl, mix the rice, pistachio
nuts and apricots. Add the remaining ingredients, toss well and season with
salt and pepper to taste.

Salsa verde

SERVES 6–8

350g (12oz) fresh flat-leafed parsley
25g (1 cup) fresh basil leaves (optional)
50g (2oz) canned anchovies
3 tbsp capers
2 garlic cloves, crushed
1 tbsp finely chopped shallots or onions
4 tbsp breadcrumbs
3–4 tbsp white wine vinegar or lemon juice
about 125ml (½ cup) olive oil

Put all the ingredients, except the olive oil, into a blender or food processor and whiz until smooth. Slowly trickle the olive oil into the mixture and gently stir to make a smooth, green sauce. If the sauce is too thick, dilute it with a little more olive oil.

Serve with raw or cooked vegetables, pasta or jacket (baked) potatoes, or spread it lightly over wholegrain bread or toast.

Smoked haddock salad

SERVES 4–6

200g (7oz) spelt or other grain, such as quinoa or wild rice, rinsed
2 naturally smoked haddock fillets
3 black peppercorns
½ onion
1 each dill and parsley sprig
½ English cucumber, chopped into small pieces

FOR THE YOGURT AND HERB DRESSING

4 tbsp Greek yogurt
2 tbsp finely chopped fresh parsley
2 tbsp finely chopped fresh dill
1 tbsp finely chopped fresh chives
½ tsp finely chopped preserved lemon or a dash of lemon juice
salt and ground black pepper

Put the spelt into a large pan of cold water and bring to the boil. Cover and simmer for 20 minutes or until cooked but not mushy. Immediately drain and rinse under cold water to prevent it from cooking further.

Put the haddock into a deep frying pan and add the peppercorns, onion and sprigs of herbs. Add cold water to just cover. Gently poach the haddock by cooking just below simmering point for 5 minutes. Remove from the pan and allow to cool.

To make the dressing, mix together the yogurt, herbs and preserved lemon. Add black pepper to taste and very little salt if needed (the haddock is already salty).

In a large bowl flake the haddock, removing any bones, and add the cucumber and spelt. Add the dressing to the haddock mixture and adjust the seasoning if necessary. Serve cold.

Carrot & spring vegetable salad

SERVES **4**

100g (¾ cup) baby carrots
200g (about 20–24) green beans
100g (heaped ¾ cup) shelled fresh broad beans
100g (⅔ cup) shelled fresh peas
150g (a large handful) mangetouts (snow peas)
100g (1 cup) baby asparagus
100g (1 bunch) each rocket (arugula) and watercress,
    divided into sprigs
a few fresh chives, roughly chopped
a few fresh basil leaves, torn
olive oil, to drizzle
a squeeze of lemon juice

FOR THE MAYONNAISE
2 egg yolks, at room temperature
1 tsp Dijon mustard
2 tbsp fresh lemon juice
ground black pepper
a pinch of salt
250ml (1 cup) olive oil

To make the mayonnaise put the egg yolks into a food processor or blender with the mustard, lemon juice, a pinch of salt and some ground black pepper. Whiz until pale and frothy, then very slowly add the oil in just a thin drizzle, whizzing slowly as you drizzle, until the mayonnaise becomes thick and glossy. Adjust the seasoning to taste and put to one side.

Steam the carrots for 6–8 minutes, then the beans, peas, mangetouts and asparagus for 3 minutes or until *al dente*. Once they're cooked, drain and rinse briefly with cold water to stop them cooking. Mix them in a bowl with the rocket and watercress. Toss in the fresh herbs, add a very light drizzle of olive oil and a squeeze of lemon juice. Serve with the mayonnaise to dip into.

Roasted aubergines with tahini

SERVES 3–4 AS A SIDE DISH, 2–3 AS A MAIN COURSE

    2 medium aubergines (eggplants),
        each cut into four lengthways
    100ml (a good ⅓ cup) olive oil
    seeds from 4 cardamom pods, ground (optional)
    25g (3 tbsp) pine nuts, toasted

FOR THE DRESSING

    2 tbsp Greek yogurt
    1 tbsp tahini
    ½ tsp very finely chopped preserved lemon,
        or lemon or lime juice to taste
    1 tbsp olive oil
    1 tsp thyme leaves
    sea salt and ground black pepper

Preheat the oven to 200°C/400°F (180°C fan oven) mark 6. Cut each piece of aubergine into three short, fat lengths. Put in a roasting tin (pan) and drizzle with the olive oil. Shake the roasting tin to ensure the aubergines are coated. Season with salt, lots of ground black pepper and the cardamom, if using. Roast for about 40–45 minutes until the aubergines are soft and toasted.

To make the dressing, mix the yogurt, tahini, preserved lemon, if using, and olive oil in a blender or use a fork or a small whisk. Season to taste with salt and black pepper and then add most of the thyme leaves. If you haven't added the preserved lemon, add a dash of lemon or lime juice and stir.

In a bowl, gently mix the aubergines into the dressing while they are still warm. Leave for 20 minutes and then serve scattered with the toasted pine nuts and the remaining thyme leaves.

Broad bean
& pistachio hummus

SERVES 4

> 1 kg (2¼lb) frozen broad beans
>   (fava beans)
> 2 tbsp shelled pistachio nuts
> leaves from 2 fresh basil sprigs
> 2 tbsp extra virgin olive oil, plus a little extra if necessary
> juice of half a lemon
> ground black pepper

Steam the broad beans for 2 minutes until they're cooked but not mushy. Rinse and cool thoroughly under cold water and remove the skins by squeezing the bean at one end – the bright green centre should just pop out.

Toast the pistachio nuts in a dry pan for 2 minutes over a gentle heat, being careful not to let them burn. Put them into a food processor or blender and blend to a fine nut powder. Add the beans and the basil, oil and lemon juice, and whiz to a mash. You can add a little extra oil or lemon juice, if you like, depending on how smooth and tart you want the hummus to be. Season with pepper.

Serve as a sandwich filling, or on jacket (baked) potatoes or pasta. Or make a delicious salad with romaine lettuce leaves, new crisp baby carrots and sliced raw vegetables, which you can dunk into the hummus.

Pan-roasted Padrón peppers

SERVES **4**

200g (7oz) small, sweet Spanish (Padrón) peppers
olive oil, for shallow frying
sea salt

Rinse the peppers and dry them. Warm a shallow pool of olive oil in a frying pan then cook the peppers over a gentle heat until they have softened. (Alternatively, roast them at 180°C/350°F (160°C fan oven) mark 4, in a baking dish with a little oil.) They will puff up and the skin will blister slightly.

Drain on kitchen paper (paper towels) and salt generously. Serve torn and added to salads or other dishes for a peppery hit.

You can buy Padrón peppers from some supermarkets or specialist delis.

Cashew
nut butter

MAKES ONE 200G (SCANT 1 CUP) JAR

200g (1⅔ cups) cashew nuts, unroasted and unsalted
3 tbsp extra virgin groundnut (peanut) or rapeseed (canola) oil
1 tsp clear honey
½ tsp sea salt

Put the nuts into a food processor and pulse until quite fine. Add 1–2 tbsp oil and process, adding more oil if needed, until you have a creamy paste. Add the honey and salt. Store in the fridge in an airtight container and use within a week.

You can also use almonds, peanuts or hazelnuts. Stir in a few chopped nuts at the end if you'd prefer a chunky butter.

Vegetable soup with lime & herbs

SERVES 4

2 garlic cloves
2 litres (8½ cups) vegetable stock
4 lemon grass stalks, bashed
5cm (2in) fresh root ginger, peeled and thinly sliced
8 lime leaves, crushed or whole
the juice of 2 limes
2 large flat (wide-capped) mushrooms, cut into thick slices
2 handfuls of frozen peas
2 handfuls of frozen broad beans
    (fava beans)
2 small hot chillies, deseeded and thinly sliced
a pinch of golden caster sugar
20 mint leaves
a large handful of coriander leaves (cilantro)

Smash the garlic to a pulp and simmer it with the stock, the lemon grass, ginger and the lime leaves for 7 minutes. Add the lime juice, mushrooms, peas, broad beans and chillies. After 2 minutes remove the lemon grass and lime leaves, and season with a pinch of sugar. Add the mint and coriander leaves.

Chicken soup

SERVES **4**

5cm (2in) piece of fresh root ginger, peeled
1 chicken, about 1.4kg (3lb)
2 celery sticks
1 medium onion
2 ripe tomatoes
2 whole star anise
6 black peppercorns
1 lime
20 mint leaves, roughly chopped
a handful of flat-leafed parsley or coriander (cilantro),
    roughly chopped
salt

Bash the ginger with a weight to crush slightly. Put the chicken into a large pan and add the celery, onion, tomatoes, ginger, 1 star anise and the peppercorns. Pour in enough water to cover. Bring to the boil briefly, then turn down the heat, cover and simmer for 1 hour.

Remove the chicken from the pan and set aside to rest. Measure out 1.4 litres (6 cups) stock and pour into a clean pan. Add the remaining star anise, the lime juice to taste and a pinch of salt. Bring to the boil and leave to simmer for 7–10 minutes. Slice the chicken breasts thinly, then put several pieces in each bowl. Spoon over the hot stock and scatter with the mint and parsley.

Oxtail soup

SERVES 4–6

1.25kg (2¾lb) oxtail, jointed and
    excess fat removed

4 tbsp plain (all-purpose) flour

about 2 tbsp olive oil

1 large carrot, roughly chopped

1 turnip, roughly chopped

1 celery stick, roughly chopped

1 large onion, roughly chopped

1 bay leaf

a few thyme sprigs

1 tsp black peppercorns

2 tsp tomato purée (tomato paste)

300ml (1¼ cups) red wine or stock

1.1 litres (4½ cups) beef stock

2 tbsp butter, softened

a handful of flat-leafed parsley,
    chopped

salt and ground black pepper

In a shallow bowl, mix 2 tbsp of the flour with salt and pepper. Heat half the oil in a large, heavy-based pan until hot. Coat the oxtail pieces with the seasoned flour, shaking off any excess, and fry for 2 minutes on each side or until evenly browned, then remove from the pan.

Add the remaining oil to the pan with the vegetables, herbs and peppercorns. Cook for 4–5 minutes until the vegetables begin to soften. Stir in the tomato purée and the remaining seasoned flour, adding a little more oil if necessary. Stir frequently for another 1–2 minutes.

Pour in the red wine and scrape the base of the pan with a wooden spoon. Boil for a few minutes. Return the oxtail to the pan and pour in the stock to cover. Bring to a simmer and skim off any scum that rises to the surface. Partially cover the pan and cook gently for 3 hours or until the oxtail is very tender and comes off the bone easily. With a pair of kitchen tongs, carefully move the oxtail pieces to a large bowl and leave to cool slightly.

Strain the cooking stock through a fine sieve (strainer) into a clean pan, pushing down on the vegetables with the back of a ladle to extract as much liquid as possible. Pull the meat from the oxtail and shred into small pieces. To thicken the stock, mix the remaining 2 tbsp of flour with the butter, then whisk into the simmering stock, a little at a time. Simmer for 5 minutes. Taste and adjust the seasoning, then add the shredded meat to the pan to warm through. Sprinkle with lots of chopped parsley before serving.

Roasted butternut squash & spicy sweetcorn soup

SERVES 4

750g (1lb 10oz) butternut squash, or
    any squash or pumpkin, cut into
    2cm (¾in) pieces
olive oil, for drizzling
1 tsp ground cumin
1 tsp ground coriander
seeds from 6 cardamom pods
25g (2 tbsp) butter
1 onion, finely chopped
2 garlic cloves, finely chopped
1 tsp turmeric
1 tsp ground ginger
2 celery sticks, finely chopped
1 leek, finely chopped
500g (1¼ cups) sweetcorn, rinsed
    and drained if canned, thawed
    if frozen
275ml (3¼ cups) semi-skimmed milk
750ml (1¼ pints) vegetable or
    chicken stock
ground black pepper
a handful of wholemeal (wholewheat)
    croutons and a swirl of natural
    (plain) yogurt, to serve (optional)

Preheat the oven to 180°C/350°F (160°C fan oven) mark 4. Put the squash on a baking tray, drizzle with olive oil and roast for 25 minutes or until golden.

Meanwhile dry-roast the cumin, coriander and cardamom seeds in a small frying pan for 2–3 minutes until they change colour and start to jump in the pan. Crush them finely, using a pestle and mortar.

Melt the butter in a large pan, then add the onion and garlic, and cook for 5 minutes or until soft. Add the ground seeds with the turmeric, ginger, celery and leek, and stir well. Cook for a further 3 minutes, then add the squash and sweetcorn. Season with black pepper. Stir well, then cover and cook over a low heat for 10 minutes. Add the milk and stock, replace the lid, bring to the boil and simmer gently for 20 minutes.

Take the soup off the heat. Whiz in a food processor or blender, leaving a little texture – it doesn't need to be absolutely smooth. Serve with wholemeal (wholewheat) bread croutons and, if you like, add a swirl of yogurt.

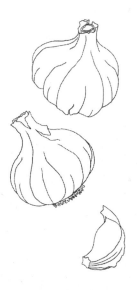

Breadsticks

MAKES 16

35g (2 tbsp or 2 cakes) fresh yeast
175ml (¾ cup) warm water
400g (3 cups) strong white (bread flour), wholemeal (wholewheat),
    Granary or spelt flour, or a combination
1 tsp salt
1 tbsp olive oil
1 tbsp fresh thyme leaves or 1 tsp dried oregano
3 tsp caraway or fennel seeds
25g (2 tbsp) butter, melted, plus extra for greasing
semolina, for dusting

Dissolve the yeast in the water, then combine it with the flour, salt and olive oil in a large bowl and mix together to make a smooth elastic dough. Knead for about 10 minutes to knock out some of the air and to develop the dough. Cover and leave to rest in a warm place for about 1 hour.

Divide the dough into two. Add the thyme leaves or dried oregano to one half and the caraway or fennel seeds to the other. Knead both balls of dough again. Roll each out into a rectangle measuring 23 x 16cm (9 x 6¼in) and cut each rectangle into eight lengths. Put the dough pieces on to a greased baking sheet, cover and leave for 10 minutes in a warm place to rise.

Meanwhile, preheat the oven to 220°C/425°F (200°C fan oven) mark 7. Brush the breadsticks with melted butter, dust with semolina and bake in the oven for 10–15 minutes until tinged golden. Transfer to a cooling rack and eat warm.

Wholemeal soda bread

MAKES AN 800G (1¾LB) LOAF

25g (2 tbsp) melted butter, plus extra for greasing
400g (3 cups) wholemeal (wholewheat) flour, plus extra for dusting
1½ tbsp caster (superfine) sugar
2 tsp bicarbonate of soda (baking soda)
½ tsp salt
225ml (1 cup) buttermilk
225ml (1 cup) water

Preheat the oven to 220°C/425°F (200°C fan oven) mark 7. Grease a
20.5cm (8in) square cake tin (pan) and dust with flour. Measure the flour into a
large bowl, then add the butter and rub it between your fingertips until evenly
dispersed. Add the sugar, bicarbonate of soda and salt, and toss this through.

In a large jug or measuring cup, measure the buttermilk and thin down with
the water. Stir this liquid through the dry ingredients quickly and evenly, then
scrape the dough into the tin and smooth it down. Place an oiled piece of foil
over the top of the tin, squeeze tightly in at the corners so that it stays in place
and bake for 20 minutes. Remove the foil.

Reduce the heat to 200°C/400°F (180°C fan oven) mark 6 and bake for a
further 10–15 minutes until brown on top. Remove from the oven and leave
to cool in the tin for 5 minutes. Take out of the tin and cool on a wire rack.

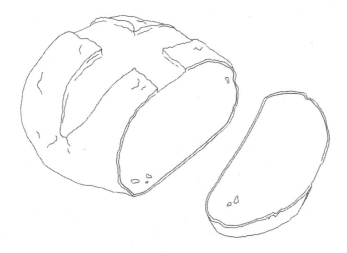

Green olive & parsley focaccia

MAKES 1 LOAF

    450g (1lb) strong bread flour, plus extra for dusting

    1½ tsp salt

    2 tsp fast-acting yeast (or a 7g (¼oz) packet)

    400ml (1¾ cups) luke-warm water

    semolina, for dusting

    a large handful of green olives, pitted and roughly chopped

    3 tbsp olive oil, plus extra for greasing

    1 garlic clove, finely chopped

    small bunch of flat-leafed parsley, chopped

    leaves from 4 thyme sprigs

    coarse sea salt

Put the flour, salt and yeast into a large bowl, mix well then pour in the water and mix to make a sticky dough. Flour the work surface generously, then turn out the dough and knead lightly for 5 minutes or until it no longer sticks to the surface. You may need to add a little more flour if the dough becomes too sticky, but it should be a little more moist than a loaf dough. Put the dough into a lightly floured bowl and cover with a tea towel or clingfilm (dishtowel or plastic wrap). Put in a warm place to rise for 1 hour or until doubled in size.

Grease a 30.5cm (12in) diameter baking tin (pan) with a little oil. Dust with a thin layer of semolina. Knock back (punch down) the dough on a floured surface for 2–3 minutes and then spread it in the baking tin. Leave to rise for 30 minutes. Preheat the oven to 220°C/425°F (200°C fan oven) mark 7.

Mix the olives with 1 tbsp oil. Stir the garlic, parsley and thyme leaves into the olives. With a floured finger, push several holes deep into the dough, then spread the olive and herb mixture over the top. Scatter with sea salt.

Bake for 25–30 minutes until pale golden, crisp on top and springy within. Drizzle with the remaining olive oil, then allow to settle. While still warm, free the bread from the pan with a palette knife, then cut or tear into pieces.

Roasted cherry tomato, basil & mozzarella pizza

SERVES **4**

> 1 quantity focaccia dough (see recipe opposite)
> oil for greasing and drizzling
> 6 canned anchovy fillets, well rinsed
> 16 ripe cherry tomatoes, halved
> 6 green or black pitted olives
> 125g (4oz) small mozzarella balls or torn mozzarella
> a few basil leaves, torn
> Parmesan cheese shavings

Make up the focaccia dough as explained in step 1 of Green olive & parsley focaccia (opposite). Roll out the dough and divide into four pieces. Roll each piece into a circle and put onto greased baking sheets. Leave to rise for 30 minutes.

Dry the anchovy fillets on kitchen paper (paper towels). Preheat the oven to 220°C/425°F (200°C fan oven) mark 7.

Gently push down the centre of the pizza base to leave about a 2.5cm (1in) rim around the edge. Scatter the cherry tomatoes over the pizza and add the anchovy fillets, olives and mozzarella on top. Finish by scattering the basil over it, then drizzle with a little olive oil. Bake for 20 minutes or until the cheese has melted and the base is crisp and golden. Serve with a few shavings of freshly grated Parmesan cheese.

You can adapt the topping by adding a tomato sauce, canned fish, such as sardines, or slices of salami or prosciutto, smoked salmon, lean ham or roast chicken. Alternatively, add steamed asparagus spears, canned artichoke hearts or sliced mushrooms.

Baked apples

- 50g (⅓ cup) sultanas (golden raisins)
- 50g (⅓ cup) dried unsulphured apricots, finely chopped
- 25g (3 tbsp) dried currants
- 25g (1oz) dried figs, stalks removed and finely chopped
- 1 tbsp pure fruit apple and pear spread
- 2 tbsp fresh orange juice
- 2 tbsp dried coconut shavings (optional)
- 4 cooking apples
- custard, natural (plain) yogurt or ice cream, to serve

Preheat the oven to 180°C/350°F (160°C fan oven) mark 4. Make the filling by putting all the ingredients, except the apples, in a bowl. Mix together, then leave for 20 minutes to allow the flavours to blend.

Core the apples, then cut them in half crossways. Put on a baking sheet, skin-side down. Stuff the mixture into the middle of the apples. The filling will also spread over the top.

Cover with foil and bake on the middle shelf of the oven for 25–30 minutes, until the apple is soft. Serve with custard, natural yogurt or ice cream.

The apples are also delicious cold and make a tasty breakfast dish.

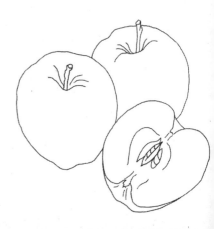

Poached rhubarb
& blueberries

SERVES **4**

250g (9oz) rhubarb
200g (7oz) blueberries
2 tbsp water
about 2 tsp maple syrup or clear honey

Preheat the oven to 170°C/350°F (150°C fan oven) mark 3. Cut the rhubarb into short lengths and put into an ovenproof dish with the blueberries. Add the water and drizzle the maple syrup over them. Stir gently and bake for 1 hour or until the fruit is soft, then taste to see if you need any more maple syrup or honey (this will depend on the sweetness of the fruit and your personal taste). Serve warm or thoroughly chilled.

Poached peaches & nectarines

SERVES 8

4 firm peaches

4 firm nectarines

75g (¼ cup) pure fruit spread, such as orange or grapefruit,
    or jam with no added sugar

4 thinly pared strips of orange rind

½ tsp rose-water (optional)

rose petals (optional)

custard or yogurt, to serve

Choose a pan large enough to fit all the fruit tightly in a single layer. Pour 600ml (2½ cups) cold water into the pan and add the fruit spread and orange rind. Gently heat until the spread has dissolved, then bring to the boil.

Carefully put the peaches and nectarines into the pan using a slotted spoon. Cover and cook for 8 minutes, turning the fruit over if it is not completely submerged in the liquid. Reduce the heat, cover and simmer gently for a further 5 minutes or until the fruit is tender.

Remove the pan from the heat and cool the fruit in the syrup for 15 minutes. Using a slotted spoon, remove the fruit and transfer to a serving dish. Set aside.

Bring the liquid in the pan to the boil and boil until it has reduced by half. Allow to cool slightly, then add the rose-water, if using, and pour the liquid over the fruit. Cool completely before serving with custard or yogurt and with rose petals, if you like.

The fruits are also good sliced over muesli, porridge or yogurt for breakfast, and can even be mashed and spread on toast.

Brown bread & hazelnut frozen yogurt

SERVES 4

- 65g (2½ oz) soft, fresh wholemeal breadcrumbs
- 65g (⅓ cup) light muscovado sugar
- 65g (⅓ cup) golden caster sugar
- 100g (¾ cup) skinned hazelnuts
- 100ml (⅓ cup) double (heavy) cream
- 400ml (1¾ cups) Greek yogurt

Put the breadcrumbs in a bowl and add the sugars. Whiz the hazelnuts in a food processor or nut mill until they are like coarse gravel, or chop them finely by hand. Thoroughly mix the nuts into the breadcrumbs and sugar, then spread out in a shallow layer over a baking tray. Put under a hot grill (broiler) and grill (broil) until the sugar, nuts and crumbs are deep golden – be careful, as the sugar can burn very easily. Leave to cool then break up into small pieces.

Mix the cream and yogurt together in a bowl. Add the sugared crumbs and stir well.

Using an ice cream maker: pour into the ice cream maker and churn until frozen, then transfer to a freezerproof container and freeze until needed.

To make by hand: put the mixture into a freezerproof container and freeze for 1–2 hours until it starts to form crystals around the edges. Stir well, using a fork, to break up the crystals, and freeze again. Repeat twice more, then leave to freeze until needed.

Before serving, take the yogurt out of the freezer and allow it to soften a little.

A little cream gives a frozen yogurt a good texture, but if you want to reduce the fat content use 500ml (2⅓ cups) yogurt and omit the cream.

Frozen raspberry & blackberry yogurt

SERVES 4

> 100g (¾ cup) raspberries
> 50g (heaped ⅓ cup) blackberries
> 1 tbsp apple concentrate
> 400ml (1¾ cups) Greek yogurt
> 3 tbsp double (heavy) cream
> 1 tsp vanilla extract

Using an ice cream maker: whiz the berries with the apple concentrate in a blender to make a purée, then pour into the ice cream maker, with the yogurt, cream and vanilla extract. Churn until frozen, then transfer to a freezerproof container and freeze until needed.

To make by hand: mix the yogurt with the cream and vanilla extract. Put in a freezerproof container and freeze for 30 minutes.

Meanwhile, whiz the berries with the apple concentrate in a blender to make a purée. Take the yogurt mixture out of the freezer and stir well with a fork to break up the forming ice crystals. Mix in the fruit purée. Freeze for another 1–2 hours until it starts to form crystals around the edges. Stir with a fork, freeze for 2 hours and stir once more, then leave to freeze until needed.

Before serving, take the yogurt out of the freezer and allow it to soften a little.

Maya's chocolate brownies

MAKES 8–10

300g (1½ cups) golden caster sugar
250g (1 cup plus 2 tbsp) unsalted butter
250g (9oz) plain chocolate with 70% cocoa solids
4 large eggs
65g (½ cup) plain wholemeal (wholewheat) flour
65g (⅔ cup) good-quality cocoa powder
½ tsp baking powder
a pinch of salt

Preheat the oven to 180°C/350°F (160°C fan oven) mark 4. Line a 23cm (9in) square baking tin (pan) with baking parchment. Put the sugar and butter into a large bowl and beat, using an electric whisk (beater), until the mixture turns soft, white and fluffy. Break the chocolate into pieces and set 50g (½ cup) to one side. Put the remainder into another large bowl set over a pan of gently simmering water (or into top of double broiler). Leave until the chocolate has melted – do not let the water touch the base of the bowl or boil over. Meanwhile, chop the reserved chocolate into very small pieces. Take the melted chocolate off the heat and add the chocolate chunks.

Break the eggs into a small bowl and beat them lightly with a fork. Sift together the flour, cocoa powder, baking powder and salt. Add the beaten eggs, little by little, to the chocolate mixture, mixing well between additions, and continue until you have added all the egg and you have a mixture similar to chocolate custard. Using a metal spoon, gently fold in the flour and cocoa.

Spoon the brownie mixture into the prepared tin, smooth over the top and bake for 30 minutes. The top will rise slightly and the cake will appear slightly softer in the middle than around the edges. Pierce the middle of the cake with a skewer; it should come out sticky, but the mixture shouldn't be uncooked. If necessary, put the cake back into the oven for another 3–5 minutes. Leave to cool in the tin then turn out and cut into squares. (Alternatively, serve them hot from the oven with ice cream, yogurt or crème fraîche.)

Raspberry baskets

SERVES 4

450g (1lb) raspberries
1 tbsp elderflower cordial (syrup)
6 sheets of filo pastry (phyllo dough), thawed if frozen
25g (2 tbsp) butter, melted, plus extra for greasing
50ml (¼ cup) whipping cream
50ml (¼ cup) Greek yogurt
icing (confectioners') sugar, for dusting

Preheat the oven to 200°C/400°F (180°C fan oven) mark 6. Put the raspberries in a bowl and drizzle with the elderflower cordial. Lightly mix and leave to infuse while you make the baskets. Cut the filo pastry sheets in half to form 12 squares. Put four small upturned ramekin dishes (custard cups) on to a large, greased baking sheet and brush them with a little of the melted butter.

Brush 3 squares of the filo pastry with melted butter. Place 1 sheet, butter-side up, over a ramekin, pressing it down the sides. Add the other 2 sheets at different angles to form a basket. Repeat with the remaining ramekins, pastry squares and butter to make three more baskets. Bake for 8 minutes or until they turn golden. Leave the baskets to cool slightly before carefully removing them from the ramekins.

Whip the cream until thick and stir in the yogurt. Divide between the baskets. Top with the raspberries, and drizzle with the raspberry juice from the bowl. Lightly dust with a little icing sugar just before serving.

Use Greek yogurt and omit the cream, if you want to keep the fat and calorie content down.

Use any other berry if you prefer, or add a spoonful of stewed fruit.

Easy apple &
greengage strudel

SERVES 4–6

    75g (1/3 cup) butter, plus extra for greasing
    1kg (2¼ lb) cooking or tart eating apples, peeled, cored and
        finely sliced
    250g (9oz) greengages or other plums, halved and
        stones (pits) removed
    2 tbsp sultanas (golden raisins)
    1 tbsp slivered, toasted almonds
    finely grated zest and juice of ½ lemon
    2 tbsp clear honey
    1 tsp ground cinnamon
    2 tbsp wholemeal (wholewheat) breadcrumbs
    flour, for dusting
    1 packet, about 350g (12oz) filo pastry (phyllo dough),
        thawed if frozen
    icing (confectioners') sugar, for dusting

Preheat the oven to 200°C/400°F (180°C fan oven) mark 6. Butter a large
baking sheet. Put the apples, greengages, sultanas and almonds into a bowl
and add the lemon zest and juice, honey and cinnamon. Mix until the apple
slices are completely coated with honey.

Melt 25g (1oz) butter in a pan and fry the breadcrumbs until crisp. Set aside.
Melt the remaining butter. Lay out a clean tea towel (dishtowel), dust lightly
with flour and cover with a layer of filo to form a rectangle about 40.5 ×
60cm (16 × 24in) – join two sheets by overlapping them slightly if
necessary. Brush with butter, cover with another layer of filo and sprinkle with
breadcrumbs. Spread the filling along a long edge, leaving a margin at
each end. Tuck the ends over the filling. Pick up the two corners of the cloth
nearest to the filling and roll the strudel away from you, allowing it to curl
over itself.

Put the strudel on the baking sheet. Brush with a little more butter and sprinkle
with a few drops of water. Bake for 40 minutes or until crisp and golden
brown and the apple filling is soft – test by inserting a skewer. Dust with icing
sugar and serve warm, with custard, yogurt or cream.

More-ish nutty biscuits

- 100g (½ cup minus 1 tbsp) butter, at room temperature
- 50g (¼ cup) light muscovado (light brown) sugar
- 50g (¼ cup) golden caster (superfine) sugar
- 100g (½ cup minus 1 tbsp) cashew or peanut butter
- 25g (¼ cup) salted, roasted cashew nuts, roughly chopped
- 25g (¼ cup) unsalted peanuts, roughly chopped
- 100g (¾ cup) plain wholemeal (wholewheat) flour
- ½ tsp bicarbonate of soda (baking powder)
- ½ tsp baking powder

Preheat the oven to 190°C/375°F (170°C fan oven) mark 5. Line a baking sheet with baking parchment. Beat the butter and sugars together using a food processor or electric whisk (beater) until the mixture becomes pale and smooth. Mix the nut butter into the butter and sugar mixture with most of the nuts, holding back a handful or two.

Sift the flour, bicarbonate of soda and baking powder over the mixture, and stir gently to form a soft dough. Spoon heaped tablespoonfuls of the dough on to the lined baking sheet. Flatten each mound slightly.

Scatter over the remaining nuts and bake for 12–14 minutes until the biscuits (cookies) are pale golden and dry on top – they should be slightly moist inside. Cool slightly on the baking sheet, then transfer to a cooling rack to cool completely.

Although best eaten fresh, these biscuits will keep for 2–3 days in an airtight tin.

You can use any combination of chopped nuts and nut butters. If you're watching your salt intake, you can use unsalted nuts and butters. The salted nuts contrast well with the sweetness here – I don't think we should be afraid of using a little salt in home cooking.

Blackberry & apple crumble cake

SERVES 8

- 150g (²/₃ cup) butter, softened, plus extra for greasing
- 150g (¾ cup) caster sugar
- 3 large eggs
- 75g (½ cup plus 1 tbsp) plain white flour
- 1½ tsp baking powder
- 100g (1 cup) ground almonds
- 1 cooking apple, cored, quartered and thinly sliced
- 150g (1 heaped cup) frozen blackberries

FOR THE TOPPING

- 100g (½ cup minus 1 tbsp) cold butter, straight from the fridge
- 50g (¹/₃ cup plus 1 tbsp) plain (all-purpose) white flour
- 50g (¹/₃ cup plus 1 tbsp) plain wholemeal (wholewheat) flour
- 100g (½ cup) demerara sugar (raw sugar)
- 2 tbsp whole rolled oats
- icing (confectioners') sugar, for dusting

Preheat the oven to 180°C/350°F (160°C fan oven) mark 4. Grease and line a 20.5cm (8in) loose-based springform cake tin (pan), 6.5cm (2½ in) deep, with baking parchment. Beat the butter and sugar together until the mixture becomes pale, smooth and fluffy. Lightly beat the eggs, then add them gradually to the butter and sugar mixture, beating briefly after each addition. If the mixture starts to curdle, stir in 1 tbsp flour. Sieve (sift) the flour and baking powder over the mixture and fold in using a metal spoon. Fold in the almonds.

Spoon the mixture into the cake tin and smooth the top. Arrange the apple slices on top of the cake, pressing them down slightly. Scatter the blackberries over them.

To make the topping, rub the butter into the flours, then stir in the sugar and oats. Sprinkle the crumble over the top of the cake. Bake for 1 hour, then insert a skewer into the centre. It will be wet from the fruit but with no cake mixture stuck to it. Leave to cool, then dust with icing sugar.

Lemon polenta cake

SERVES 8

3 large eggs, separated
100g (½ cup) golden caster (superfine) sugar
zest and juice of 1 lemon
50g (⅓ cup) fine polenta (cornmeal)
25g (¼ cup) ground almonds

FOR THE FILLING (OPTIONAL)

125g (4oz) mascarpone cheese
2 tsp orange juice
½ tsp orange zest
1 tbsp natural (plain) yogurt
½ tbsp maple syrup

Preheat the oven to 180°C/350°F (160°C fan oven) mark 4. Grease and line a 20.5cm (8in) cake tin (pan) then lightly butter the base. Using a food processor or electric whisk (beater), beat the egg yolks and the sugar at high speed until they turn pale, thick and creamy. Gradually add the lemon juice to the creamed mixture, beating until it starts to thicken.

Mix the lemon zest, polenta and ground almonds together and stir them into the egg and sugar mixture. In a clean bowl beat the egg whites until almost stiff. Fold the egg yolk mixture into the whites using a metal spoon. Transfer the mixture to the lined cake tin and bake for 30 minutes or until the centre is cooked and the top is lightly browned. Insert a skewer into the centre – it should come out clean. Using a palette knife (or spatula), turn the cake out on to a cake rack and leave to cool.

Cut the cake in half horizontally if you want to fill it. Put the bottom half on a cake plate. To make the filling, beat the mascarpone in a bowl. Add the orange juice, zest, yogurt and maple syrup, and beat until smooth. Spread this over the cake and replace the top half, or spread half the filling over it and use the other half to top the cake.

Damson, pear & walnut muffins

MAKES 12 LARGE MUFFINS

- 25g (2 tbsp) vegetable oil, such as rapeseed (canola) or groundnut (peanut) oil, plus extra for greasing
- 150g (5oz) unsweetened breakfast flakes (such as buckwheat and rice cereal flakes, or oats and a bran-type flake)
- 150g (1 cup plus 2 tbsp) plain white (all-purpose) flour
- 100g (¾ cup) plain wholemeal (wholewheat) flour
- 125g (scant ⅔ cup) golden caster (superfine) sugar
- 1 tsp ground allspice
- 25g (¼ cup) walnuts, chopped
- 1 tsp baking powder
- a pinch of salt
- 150g (heaped ⅔ cup) natural (plain) yogurt
- 50ml (¼ cup) milk
- 2 large eggs
- 1 large firm pear (or 2 small pears)
- 200g (7oz) damson plums (fresh or frozen), stones (pits) removed and cut into eighths

Preheat the oven to 200°C/400°F (180°C fan oven) mark 6. Grease a 12-cup muffin tray. Combine the cereal flakes and dry ingredients in a large bowl. Gently combine the yogurt, milk, oil and eggs in a second bowl, using a fork.

Grate the pear and squeeze out and discard any excess liquid. Add the pear and damson slices to the dry ingredients. Pour the oil mixture into the fruit and dry ingredients and combine gently, but thoroughly, with a metal spoon. Do not overmix – use big scooping movements to mix well without beating.

Divide the mixture equally among the muffin cases. Bake for 20 minutes, then reduce the oven temperature to 180°C/350°F (160°C fan oven) mark 4 and bake for a further 10 minutes until firm and lightly golden.

Fruity beetroot cake

SERVES 8–10

- 150g (1 cup plus 2 tbsp) white self-raising flour
- 75g (½ cup plus 2 tbsp) wholemeal (wholewheat) self-raising flour
- ½ tsp bicarbonate of soda (baking soda)
- 1 tsp baking powder
- ½ tsp ground cinnamon
- 175ml (¾ cup) rapeseed (canola) or sunflower oil
- 225g (1 cup plus 2 tbsp) light muscovado (light brown) sugar
- 3 eggs, separated
- 150g (5oz) raw beetroot (beets), coarsely grated
- juice of ½ lemon
- 75g (½ cup) sultanas (golden raisins)
- 75g (½ cup) mixed seeds, such as pumpkin sunflower, hemp or linseeds (flaxseeds)

Preheat the oven to 180°C/350°F (160°C fan oven) mark 4. Lightly butter a 20.5 x 9 x 7cm (8 x 3½ x 3in) loaf tin (pan) and line the base with baking parchment.

Sift together the flours, bicarbonate of soda (baking soda), baking powder and cinnamon into a large bowl, then tip the bran left in the sieve (sifter) into the bowl (if you want to keep it).

In another bowl, beat the oil and sugar using a food processor or electric whisk (beater) until well combined. Gradually beat the egg yolks into the oil mixture.

Fold the beetroot into the mixture, then add the lemon juice, sultanas and seeds. Fold the flours and raising agents into the mixture while beating slowly.

In a clean bowl, whisk the egg whites until light and almost stiff. Fold gently into the mixture using a large metal spoon. Pour the mixture into the cake tin and bake for 50–55 minutes until risen and firm, covering the top with a piece of foil after 30 minutes. Insert a skewer into the centre – the cake should be moist inside but not sticky. Leave to cool in the tin for 20 minutes, then remove from the tin and cool completely on a cooling rack.

Index

About the author

Jane Clarke, BSc (Honours) SRD, is Britain's most trusted nutritionist and a trained Cordon Bleu chef, whose belief is grounded in the simple statement that 'food nourishes your life, not just your body'. Jane's mission is to change people's lives through the power of nourishment and she has pursued this ambition through her extensive writing, TV presenting, personal appearances, charity work and private practices.

One of the most influential health writers in the UK and Europe today, Jane is also a qualified dietician. She continues to spearhead nutrition practices, including a specialist Oncology Nutrition Practice in Marylebone, London, advising some of Britain's leading professional sportspeople and many of the world's biggest music and media personalities, whilst also treating young children and the elderly with health problems such as diabetes and dementia.

Jane is the author of several best-selling books, has been a columnist for the *Daily Mail*, *The Observer*, *The Times* and the *Mail on Sunday*. Her blog and website www.janeclarke.com provides cutting-edge scoops on health stories and delicious recipes.

Acknowledgements

A large number of people have generously shared their time, knowledge and support with me in writing this book. My family continue to be amazing and I am also lucky enough to have a set of very treasured friends, who have pulled me out of writers block dips, listened to my screams as recipes have flopped and inspired me to keep going until the final page was delivered.
In particular I'd like to thank Cat Vinton, Lesja Liber, Gill and Mike Walsh, Pauline and Clive Pitts, Theodore and Ruth Gillick, Sam and David Galer-Rose, Vanessa Fairfax, Dr Martin Scurr, Professor Justin Stebbing, Jo Milloy, Katingo Giannoulis, Caroline Peppercorn, Navin Poddar, Matt Utber. I couldn't enjoy my writing and my work without such a supportive group of colleagues who in their own way point me in the right direction, in particular my agent along with Susan Hutter, Paul Chiappe, and my treasured editor Annie Lee. And when it came to turning my manuscript into a beautiful book, I want to thank Katie Cowan, Caroline King, Howard Sooley, Jane McIntosh, Jilly Sitford and Martin Topping at Ome Design, Sarah Rock, Tim Hart and his team at Hambleton Hall for the lovely location and Julian Carter for his help at Hambleton Bakery.

Picture Credits
All photography by Howard Sooley except author photograph by Cat Vinton (www.catvphotography.co.uk). Illustrations by Jilly Sitford at Ome Design (www.omedesign.co.uk.)